THE
IBS
HANDBOOK

A Guide to
Understanding and Treating
Irritable Bowel Syndrome

by
Bill Habets

First published in Great Britain MCMXCIII by Carnell plc, 28 Eccleston Square, London SW1V 1PU.

Copyright © MCMXCIII by Carnell plc.

Typeset by SJ Design and Publishing, Bromley, Kent.

Printed by Repro City Limited, London.

ISBN 1-85779-184-3

Contents

Foreword

IRRITABLE BOWEL Syndrome (IBS) has been described as 'the most miserable of all chronic diseases, not the worst, not the most dangerous, just the most miserable'.

While the quotation above may be guilty of overstating the situation somewhat, there is nevertheless little doubt that IBS can make life truly miserable for those unfortunate enough to be afflicted by it. Contributing to this misery are two major facts: first of all, sufferers are usually only too aware that medicine as a whole still remains largely ignorant about many of the basic aspects of IBS and that while treatments do offer relief, they don't provide a cure. Secondly, those who have 'moderate' IBS will often not seek out such medical help as is available.

Another one of the problems with the disorder is that its symptoms can be so vague, so sporadic, and even so conflicting, that those who experience them may not even realise for some time that these are all part of a pattern which is characteristic of IBS. It's not at all uncommon for it to take some years before someone comes to the conclusion that various bouts of quite differing digestive difficulties are all part of a larger picture.

All in all, IBS in general is quite a unique ailment. This uniqueness is further reflected in the way it manifests its symptoms in individuals with almost every case being somewhat different in presentation from others. It's not all that surprising, therefore, that a sufferer may not immediately identify the disorder that's afflicting him or her.

Whatever an individual's circumstances, there is one thing that's invariably needed – and that's information. While your doctor should always be your first source of information, there are nevertheless usually some questions that remain unanswered after a consultation, if only because of the pressure of time. It is to help fill that information gap that this book was written. It is also hoped that it will give you a better understanding of your disorder and may even assist you in dealing with it more satisfactorily.

As you read on, however, please bear two most important points in mind. *Firstly, a book like this one cannot be – nor is it intended to be – in any way a substitute for professional medical opinion. Readers are, therefore, earnestly urged always to consult their own doctor before trying out any form of therapy, starting a new diet, or engaging in what is for them a new type of physical exercise. Only your own doctor can help you decide what may or may not be helpful or appropriate in the specific circumstances of your individual case.*

Secondly, although the information offered in this book is based upon the views of doctors, specialists and other health professionals, these experts by no means always agree amongst themselves about many aspects of IBS. This means that on many subjects there are indeed dissenting opinions and whenever possible I've tried to present all sides of a particular argument.

Finally, I'd like to express my gratitude to all those who have given so generously of their time and expertise during my research. They are too many to mention individually, but to each and every one of them, my sincere and appreciative thanks.

Bill Habets

Chapter 1

What Is Irritable Bowel Syndrome?

THE PHRASE 'Irritable Bowel Syndrome' – which is rather a mouthful and therefore is generally condensed into what is known as 'IBS' – is often used rather loosely to cover a multitude of digestive problems.

Strictly speaking, however, IBS is described in most medical textbooks as a common condition which has some, if not necessarily all, of the following characteristics:

- There is recurrent pain or discomfort – this can range from mild discomfort to acute pain and this can be present all the time, some of the time, or just very occasionally. The severity of the pain can also vary greatly during various episodes.
- There is either constipation and/or diarrhoea at least some of the time.
- There is no structural – that is organic – disease present that can be detected.
- The symptoms are usually the result of abnormal contractions in the colon.
- The condition is usually chronic in that it can continue without much overall change in the symptoms for many years.
- Although the condition may last for years, it is not accompanied by any deterioration in the general health of the sufferer, except perhaps for that which may be caused by the psychological effects of suffering the condition rather than any due to the disorder itself.
- The cause of the condition remains unknown, but it is often associated with either stress or anxiety and it is likely that it first

arose following a severe infection of the intestine.

☐ Treatment is usually based on one or more of the following four major approaches: by dietary adjustment; by removing or lessening anxiety, possibly by psychotherapy; by using faecal softening agents; or by using antispasmodic drugs.

The first thing that emerges from the above is that IBS is not a clearly-defined disease, such as, for example, appendicitis or tuberculosis. It is instead a sometimes vague catch-all phrase under which are lumped a variety of symptoms for which there otherwise seems to be no particular explanation. The inclusion of the word 'syndrome' in the label 'IBS', of course, points to this vagueness: 'syndrome' means a combination of various signs and/or symptoms that form a distinct clinical picture that is indicative of a particular disorder. The key word in that last definition is, of course, 'indicative', meaning that it points to and suggests that a particular disorder may be the cause of the symptoms, but that this is merely *indicated* and certainly not fully proven to be so.

While it may be difficult to pin down with exactitude what is and what isn't IBS, this strangely enough is perhaps not all that important much of the time. This is because treatment is often based on the very pragmatic view that if the patient responds well to something that is meant to alleviate IBS, well then, it must have been IBS he or she had in the first instance.

Although medical experts may differ on the exact definition of IBS, this can be likened to theologians arguing about how many angels can dance on the head of a pin – it's interesting stuff for a discussion, but not all that relevant to everyday life. What is relevant, however, as far as IBS is concerned, is what can be done about relieving the suffering of the many millions of people who are affected by it. The good news about this is that just about everyone can expect a substantial improvement if the right treatment is obtained. What is the right treatment will vary considerably from patient to patient and what may more or less cure IBS in one patient may not make the slightest difference for another. This highly variable response to treatment is another characteristic aspect of IBS and one that can make even retrospective diagnosis with the full benefit of hindsight still a matter for conjecture.

An alternative way of identifying other diseases is by looking at the kind of people they mainly tend to affect and then see whether or not a given patient broadly fits that profile. Once again, this method doesn't work all that well with IBS because just about anyone, no matter what his or her lifestyle, no matter what age, may have it.

So IBS is a disorder with many different kinds of symptoms – some of which can be quite contradictory in nature – and which can strike anyone. The root-causes for the symptoms remain largely unknown and treatment is frequently based on a principle which can be summed up as 'Let's try this and see if it does the trick … if it doesn't, we'll try something else'. What then is truly known for sure about this disorder?

Well, there is at least one fact about it upon which all experts agree: there are many millions of IBS sufferers in this country alone. But exactly how prevalent IBS is remains a matter of some dispute within the medical profession because this depends on how you define IBS. For example, do you include someone who just occasionally has IBS-like symptoms, but is hardly suffering badly from it? Or do you just count those who are afflicted severely enough that they seek medical help? Without widely accepted criteria, it's not surprising then that the figures from various sources may fluctuate widely. However, after collating all the best information from the most reliable sources, the following conclusions emerge:

□ It is estimated that about one third of all people get some of the symptoms of IBS some of the time.

□ About 15 per cent of the general population have the symptoms of IBS on a regular basis.

□ About half of the patients seen by gastroenterologists in hospital clinics end up being diagnosed as having IBS.

The figures quoted above are for the United Kingdom, but those for the rest of the Western world are broadly similar. So it's clear that IBS is a major world-wide problem and individual sufferers can at least find some reassurance and perhaps even comfort in the fact that they're hardly alone in having to cope with a variety of sometimes extremely unpleasant symptoms.

As far as to what kind of people get IBS is concerned, although the short answer to this question is, as seen earlier, that anyone can, it is accepted that women are much more likely to suffer from the condition than men are, *perhaps up to five times more so*. The latter is, however, based on the total of IBS sufferers actually seen by doctors and the information may be somewhat misleading in that it could be that there are many more men who don't seek help for their symptoms and whose numbers therefore remain uncounted. In fact, this same proviso needs to be applied to all figures relating to IBS incidence – many sufferers are unrecorded because they put up with the problem without looking for medical help.

It is, of course, a great shame that this should be the case as no one should resignedly be subjected to continued discomfort or pain over any length of time. Yet, experts agree that this is exactly what happens with IBS and much more so with this particular disorder than with most others.

The reasons for this marked reluctance exhibited by probably the majority of sufferers to come forward with their symptoms resides in two main factors. Firstly, the symptoms are by definition associated with problems involved with bowel movements, a subject about which there is a natural and understandable shyness or reticence. Secondly, as some of the symptoms may at times resemble those of serious organic diseases like cancer, sufferers fearing the worst but not wanting to have this confirmed simply keep on postponing the evil day when they have to admit they need help. It should go without saying – but it won't – that neither of these reasons are good ones and that everyone who has symptoms of any severity whatsoever should consult his or her doctor about them, if only for the reassurance that this may bring.

The other problem with getting to grips with who does and doesn't have IBS is that the symptoms often come and go without any identifiable reason. This means that many a sufferer – who would be medically diagnosed as having IBS – may simply ignore the temporary problems caused by the disorder, ascribing them to various other factors, such as having had a meal that was too spicy or having experienced a tense day at work.

Summing up the above, we find that:

□ IBS is a condition which is poorly defined and, to use the colloquial phrase, 'covers a multitude of sins'.

□ Something like about half of us have it at one time or another in our lives.

□ Most of those who suffer from it will not seek medical advice.

That, in a sense, is the bad news about IBS. Now for the good news:

□ If you have IBS, you can almost certainly control it to such an extent that it will be, broadly speaking, non-existent as far as its symptoms are concerned. This doesn't mean that you've necessarily been cured of the underlying disorder, just that it won't bother you – this, of course, being to all extents and purposes nearly as good as a cure as far as most people are concerned.

□ Even if you choose not to do anything about your problems – providing they are truly caused by IBS and not by something else provoking similar symptoms – the chances are that they won't get any worse and certainly won't kill or incapacitate you in the end.

□ A vast amount of research is being done about how to treat IBS and while so far this has provided but comparatively little positive information, the experts agree that the day of the big breakthrough must now be very close at hand.

□ Although it's obvious that your first source of help and advice should always be your doctor, IBS is one of those complaints which often respond extremely well to some very simple self-help measures. It may well be that all you need to do to overcome your IBS is to follow some very basic dietary guidelines.

Controlling what you eat is, of course, one of the main approaches to treatment and this can very frequently bring about drastic improvements in a very short period of time. A dramatic instance of this was recounted in a recent edition of *Gastroenterology in Practice* in which Dr Elizabeth Scott, who has a special interest in IBS, told the story of a patient who had been troubled with severe symptoms for years. When the patient was asked to describe a typical day's intake of food, this is what the doctor was told: "Breakfast, one can of coke; mid-morning snack, two cans of coke and a packet of crisps; lunch, one can of coke and two packets of crisps; dinner, microchips, peas and a tin of soup." The treatment was obvious and Dr Scott wryly commented: "The patient was cured by introducing a balanced diet."

The above is not meant to suggest that either identifying what's causing the problem or eliminating its cause is always that easy. It does, however, show that a careful assessment of the various aspects of a sufferer's lifestyle will often point the way to what is amiss and how this can be corrected.

That is what this book is all about – providing you with all the relevant information you need so that working together with your doctor you can help yourself and thereby eliminate all your troublesome symptoms.

As you read on, it's worth keeping in mind that although the name of the disorder is 'Irritable Bowel Syndrome', the roots of your difficulties may often lie elsewhere than in the bowel itself and that your IBS symptoms may be merely a reflection of what's wrong elsewhere. However, as most of the identifiable symptoms do arise in the digestive system, we will begin by looking at this in some detail in the next chapter.

Chapter 2

A Tour Of The Digestive System

A S WAS indicated at the end of the previous chapter, while the symptoms of Irritable Bowel Syndrome are usually primarily linked to the bowel, some of these can result from problems in other parts of the digestive system. It is, therefore, just as well to become acquainted with the various organs which make up this system and how they interact.

Before that, however, a brief look at what exactly is meant by the word 'bowel'....

This word can be used interchangeably with either 'intestine' or 'gut' to describe that part of the alimentary canal that extends from the stomach to the anus and divides into two main parts:

1)   The *small intestine*, which in turn is divided into the duodenum, the jejunum, and the ileum;

2)   The *large intestine*, consisting of the caecum, the vermiform appendix, the colon, and the rectum.

By the way, it is worth noting in this context that the word 'gut' is not as some might suppose a vulgar or vernacular alternative to 'bowel', but is instead a perfectly acceptable and descriptive term, being defined in the Concise Oxford Dictionary as a 'particular part of the lower alimentary canal'. Incidentally, in medical usage the word takes the singular form, not the plural which is how it is often used in everyday language.

While on the subject of words and their meaning, it might be just as well to define 'digestion': in a medical context, this means the process which breaks down insoluble food consisting of large molecules, into soluble compounds consisting of smaller molecules. Although most of this process takes place in the stomach and small intestine, it also involves other parts of the alimentary canal, including the mouth. Then there's 'ingestion', which simply describes the act of taking food through the mouth, and 'absorption' which defines the uptake of fluids and other substances by the tissues of the body. Absorption is followed by 'assimilation', the name given to the process by which food substances are taken into the cells of the body after having first undergone digestion and absorption. Finally, there's 'egestion' which means the expulsion of undigested remains of food from the alimentary canal.

Let us now set out on a guided tour of the alimentary canal and see how and where these various processes occur and work together.

THE MOUTH

The digestive process is started logically enough by the act of ingesting food, that is putting it in your mouth where two very important actions take place:

1) First of all, biting and chewing the food reduces it to pieces of a size suitable for eventual swallowing. But there's more to chewing than merely making the morsels of food smaller. By chewing you also automatically increase the total surface of the food and this greatly affects the efficiency of the second process which is simultaneously at work in the mouth.

2) While the food is being chewed it is also being mixed with saliva, this being the digestive juice which is secreted by the salivary glands whose ducts lead into the mouth. There are three pairs of these glands: the *parotid glands* – these are located in front of each ear and their ducts (known as Stensen's ducts) terminate on the inner side of the cheeks, opposite the second upper molar teeth; the *sublingual glands* – located in the lower part of the

mouth, one on each side of the tongue, and each with about 20 ducts which lead directly into the mouth above the glands; and the *submandibular glands*, which are situated below the parotid glands whose ducts (called Wharton's ducts) open under the tongue. These glands have two different types of cells – one type produces *mucus* and the other a special enzyme called *salivary amylase* which combine to create saliva.

Before proceeding further, a brief word about enzymes as we shall be encountering these time and time again in other parts of the digestive system.

Broadly speaking, enzymes are chemical compounds which are protein in nature and which are manufactured in the cells of living organisms. In small amounts, enzymes act as catalysts, that is they speed up the rate of a biological reaction without themselves being used up in the reaction. There are many different kinds of enzymes because each is relatively specific in the kind of reaction it catalyses as will be seen later when the specific enzymes to be found in the various digestive juices will be identified.

In the instance of the mouth, at the very starting point of the digestive system, food then first comes into contact with the 'digestive juice' called saliva and the enzyme in that juice is 'salivary amylase'. This is usually slightly acid and acts upon starch to produce maltose, a sugar consisting of two molecules of glucose.

Unlike most other digestive juices which are only secreted when food is present in the relevant part of the alimentary canal so as to prevent wasting enzymes, saliva is secreted continuously because it has other tasks to perform apart from aiding digestion. These include promoting cleanliness in the mouth even when no food is being ingested and also permitting clear speech by keeping the lining of the mouth moist. The amount of saliva being produced does, however, increase dramatically during ingestion and the salivary glands are also stimulated by reflex action initiated by the taste, smell, sight or even the mere thought of food.

As food in the mouth is being chewed and ground by the teeth – the process known as *mastication* – the mucus in the saliva lubricates the food and at the same time helps to stick the particles together. Simultaneously, the salivary amylase acts on starch within the food. It's obvious therefore that the longer the food is retained in the mouth the greater will be this action of starch digestion. Another important role performed by saliva is that it dissolves small amounts of the food thereby stimulating the taste-sensitive cells in the tongue.

THE OESOPHAGUS

When the food has been reduced to small enough morsels, it is eventually swallowed, as a pellet of food – now known as a 'bolus' – is pressed by the tongue to the back of the mouth. Swallowing starts as a voluntary action, but becomes a reflex – or automatic – action once the bolus reaches what is in effect a point of no return. Having passed through the back of the mouth (the pharynx), the bolus is directed by the epiglottis, a flap of cartilage, to travel over the tracheal opening without entering it and then enters the oesophagus (or gullet). Depending upon its consistency, the food will take about six seconds to descend down the gullet into the stomach. Liquids, of course, will travel the same distance in a much shorter period of time.

The passage of food down the gullet is aided by a mechanism known as *peristalsis* which is to be found at work in other parts of the alimentary canal. Peristalsis is a wave-like movement that progresses along many of the hollow tubes in the human body. It occurs automatically as needed and is characteristically found in tubes that have both circular and longitudinal muscle fibres. By alternatively contracting and relaxing, the circular muscles propel the food forward in a wave-like motion.

THE STOMACH

This is a distensible sack-like organ, lying just below the diaphragm, to the right of the spleen and partially under the liver. It is connected to the oesophagus via the *cardiac orifice* at the top and to the duodenum through the *pyloric sphincter* below.

The walls of the stomach are very elastic and so it can extend itself to hold comfortably quite large quantities of food which are retained within it by the closing of the pyloric sphincter. One of the functions of the stomach is to provide a holding stage where food from a meal can be stored and gradually released to the rest of the alimentary canal.

Little absorption of food actually takes place in the stomach, except for water, some salts, a little glucose and alcohol. However, numerous tube-like glands in the lining of the stomach do produce gastric juice which contains a vital enzyme known as *pepsin* which acts upon proteins to produce *peptides*, these being molecules consisting of two or more amino acids. In young children, gastric juice may also contain a second enzyme known as *rennin* whose job it is to clot milk protein.

The gastric juices and the food are churned up in the stomach by rhythmic peristaltic waves which travel from the cardiac orifice to the pyloric sphincter every twenty seconds or so. This churning eventually reduces the food to a cream-like fluid known as *chyme* and it is this which in turn is expelled from the stomach into the duodenum.

How long a given food may be retained in the stomach varies considerably, but typically a mainly starch meal such as porridge may take an hour or somewhat less to pass through while meat will take perhaps two or three times as long. Water and other liquids may travel though the stomach in a matter of minutes. On the other hand, fatty foods will slow down the rate at which the stomach empties itself.

Apart from the type of food it's dealing with, the stomach's retention of it can also be affected by outside factors. For example, fear may reduce gastric movement while excitement will generally hasten it.

The secretion of the stomach's digestive juice is set off automatically as it responds to the presence of food in the mouth and once initiated it is then maintained as long as food, especially meat, remains in the stomach. Food also liberates a special hormone – called *gastrin* – from the pyloric end of the stomach and this hormone stimulates the ongoing production of enzymes by the gastric glands.

THE DUODENUM

This is the first of the three separate parts that make up the small intestine – which incidentally is called so because on the average it is just over an inch, that is about three centimetres, in diameter, although its total length is about twenty feet, or about six metres – and extends from the pylorus of the stomach to the jejunum. The main purpose of the duodenum is to act as a sort of mixing chamber where the food which has come down from the stomach is subjected to more digestive juices, which in this instance originate from the pancreas and the liver.

☐ From the pancreas, which is a cream-coloured gland lying below the stomach, comes some 1,500 cubic centimetres of *pancreatic juice* every day and this contains water, sodium hydrogencarbonate and three enzymes: an amylase which acts on starch; a lipase which acts on fats; and 'trypsinogen' which remains inactive until it is combined with a chemical activator secreted by the mucosa of the duodenum and is then transformed into the enzyme 'trypsin', which breaks down proteins into peptides. The purpose of the sodium hydrogencarbonate in the pancreatic juice is to reduce the acidity of the chyme, thereby creating an environment with a suitable pH for both the pancreatic and intestinal enzymes.

☐ From the liver – via the gall-bladder – comes *bile*, which is a greenish, watery, alkaline fluid which is manufactured continuously in the liver at the rate of between 500 to 1,000 cubic centimetres a day. The bile is stored until required in the gall-bladder where it is also made into a concentration that is about ten times stronger. The addition of the bile to the chyme in the duodenum fulfils two tasks: first of all, it emulsifies fats; and secondly, it aids their absorption which is most important because any disorder which adversely affects the absorption of fats also automatically thereby impairs the uptake of vitamins A, D and K, which are fat-soluble.

The duodenum is comparatively short and is usually less than a foot in length. It is, of course, the site where duodenal ulcers occur and as the pain created by these can sometimes be confused with the symptoms of irritable bowel syndrome, it may be best to interrupt our voyage through the alimentary canal temporarily and briefly consider this ailment.

A duodenal ulcer is usually the result of the action of acid and pepsin on the mucosa, that is the lining, of the duodenum of a predisposed individual. An increased output of stomach acid is frequently the root-cause and for no discernible reason this is more likely to occur in people whose blood is in group O. Common symptoms of a duodenal ulcer include: pain in the upper abdomen, this happening more frequently when the stomach is relatively empty; and vomiting. The symptoms are frequently relieved by antacid medication or surgery may be needed if complications – such as perforation or obstruction – ensue. A duodenal ulcer is a complaint quite separate from IBS and its existence can normally be established without difficulty.

Continuing our journey along the alimentary canal, we now find that the food after leaving the duodenum enters the second part of the small intestine, the ileum.

THE ILEUM

Although the small intestine is correctly divided into three sections – the duodenum, as described above, the jejunum and the ileum – as far as studying the process of digestion is concerned we can, in effect, lump the jejunum and ileum together and cover both of these under the single term 'ileum'. For those who are interested, the jejunum is, technically speaking, that part of the small intestine which links the duodenum to the ileum proper.

Food passing through the ileum is subjected to a new gastric juice – called *succus entericus* – which comes from glands located in the lining of the ileum. Succus entericus contains the following enzymes:

1) *Erepsin* which acts upon peptides to produce amino acids;

2) *Lipase* which acts upon fats to produce fatty acids and glycerol;

3) *Sucrase* which acts upon sucrose to produce glucose and fructose;

4) *Lactase* which acts upon lactose to produce glucose and galactose;

5) *Maltase* which acts upon maltose to produce glucose.

The ileum is the region of the alimentary canal where nearly all of the absorption of digested food takes place as most of the digestible material has by now been reduced into soluble compounds which can be transferred into the blood stream through the intestinal lining. To aid in this process of absorption, the ileum has several characteristic properties:

- It is very long – and therefore it offers a very large surface through which the digested food can be absorbed.

- Large though this surface is, it is further augmented by many thousands of extremely small projections called *villi* (singular: villus) of which there are about 30 to each square millimetre.

- The *epithelium* – that is the tissue that lines the ileum – is extremely thin and this makes it possible for fluid to pass through it both rapidly and efficiently. Absorption occurs as the molecules of amino acids and glucose pass though this lining and the walls of the capillaries to enter the blood plasma.

The food residue – depending upon what it was originally – may spend some three to four hours in the small intestine before it travels via the *ileo-colic sphincter* to enter the large intestine.

THE LARGE INTESTINE

The starting point of the large intestine is quite low down on the right side of your abdomen and, as its name suggests, it is much larger in diameter than the small intestine, being about two and a half inches (or about 6 centimetres) wide. It is, however, comparatively short and its average length is about five feet (about a metre and a half).

The large intestine divides into several parts:

□ First of all, there is the *colon* itself which forms the largest unit, a kind of upside down U-shape which begins at the lower right of the abdomen and travels upwards, then across the belly, and eventually descends down the left side of the body. Each section of the colon has its own name: the first part at the right side is known, quite reasonably, as the *ascending colon*; that which crosses the body more or less horizontally is called the *transverse colon*; and that which goes back down again is known, as might have been expected, as the *descending colon*. Finally there is the *sigmoid colon*, which is the S-shaped terminal part of the descending colon that leads to the rectum. There are also special names for the bends in the colon – the one at the top of the ascending colon is called the *repatic flexure* and the one at the end of the transverse colon is known as the *solenic flexure*.

□ Other parts of the large intestine are the *caecum*, a blind-ended pouch which hangs below the junction of the large and small intestines, and the *vermiform appendix*, a short blind-ended tube that is attached to the end of the caecum. The functions of both the appendix and the caecum in man are unclear, although they play an important role in the digestive system of herbivores as they are the sites in which much of the cellulose digestion takes place. The appendix, of course, is well-known for its tendency to become infected or inflamed, a condition known as appendicitis which is treated by surgical removal of the appendix.

□ The *rectum* is the final part of the large intestine and is usually about five inches (12 centimetres) long and runs from the sigmoid colon to the anal canal. It serves as a storage area for faeces before they are eliminated.

Little – if any – absorption of food takes place in the large intestine and the material passing into it from the small intestine consists primarily of water and undigested matter. This is made up mainly of vegetable fibres – that is 'roughage' – as well as cellulose, dead bacteria, mucus, salts and dead cells that became loosened from the lining of the alimentary canal.

One of the colon's major functions is to allow the absorption of much of the water from the undigested residue. This is a vital task because the secretion of the various digestive juices takes a large amount of water from the body and, were this not returned to it in due course, this could easily lead to dehydration.

Dehydration is in fact one of the main problems that diarrhoea may present because when that happens the contents of the colon are expelled long before adequate absorption of water has had the chance to take place. And if the diarrhoea is severe and prolonged, it can also lead to excess losses of salts and nutrients in the faeces.

Under normal circumstances, however, the food residues spend something like 12 to 24 hours in the large intestine, gradually being moved along by peristaltic waves every few hours to be eventually propelled into the rectum.

The above is, of course, a simplified description of the digestive system, but it nevertheless does indicate the main components and how they have to work together smoothly to provide trouble-free digestion. It is not surprising, however, that when things go wrong, such a complicated system can create a wide variety of symptoms, many of which fall under the overall heading of 'irritable bowel syndrome'. In the next chapter, we will look at these symptoms in detail.

Chapter 3

The Symptoms Of
Irritable Bowel Syndrome

THE VERY first thing that has to be said about the term 'Irritable Bowel Syndrome' is that it is rather a misleading one that in itself can cause a great deal of confusion.

First of all, as will be explained later, it's not so much a question of the bowel being 'irritable' or even 'irritated' as the problems are much more likely to stem from one that is sluggish or lethargic, or over-active, or inconsistent in its behaviour.

Secondly, although many of the symptoms linked to IBS do seem to stem from the intestines – that is the bowel – that is by no means always the case and not infrequently the source of the problem lies elsewhere within the digestive system.

Even the word 'syndrome' – which broadly speaking means 'a combination of symptoms and/or signs that form a distinctive clinical picture indicative of a particular disorder' – is not quite correct because the picture that emerges from IBS is generally less than distinctive and often is most unclear indeed.

Satisfactory or not, IBS nevertheless is the term we're stuck with. Unfortunately, it's one that can mean many different things to different people, as we will find out. But, to begin, let us look at how it is used within a medical context when it is usually meant to describe a condition which has the following main characteristics:

1)   The patient suffers from recurrent abdominal pain;

2)   Constipation and/or diarrhoea occurs frequently over a period of many months or even years;

3) There is no detectable structural disease;
4) The symptoms are caused by abnormal muscular contractions in the colon.

If one were solely to use the above guidelines, it would be a reasonably easy task to determine what is and what isn't IBS. However, different criteria are suggested by a variety of other highly knowledgeable sources. For example, a paper published in the *British Journal of Pharmaceutical Practice* and called 'Therapeutic Options In Irritable Bowel Syndrome' which reviewed 50 consecutive IBS patients attending a gastroenterology clinic stated: 'There are at least four different patterns of clinical presentation based on the type of bowel habit experienced. These are: constipation; diarrhoea; alternating constipation and diarrhoea; and normal bowel habit.'

So the definition of IBS that seemed so straightforward at first has already been changed because it can now also include 'normal bowel habit' as well as either constipation and/or diarrhoea. This, of course, adds up to saying that bowel habit by itself and whether normal or not is not necessarily any indication whatever of IBS. Despite that, it's obvious that in most cases there is evidence of bowel habit that is not normal. For example, looking at the 50 patients – of which 43 were females and 7 males, ranging in age from 21 to 60 years, with more than two thirds under the age of 40 – involved in the study mentioned earlier we find that:

□ The most common form of IBS was alternating constipation and diarrhoea and this accounted for 44 per cent of those interviewed.
□ The next most prevalent form of IBS was constipation and this was how 36 per cent of the cases presented themselves.
□ Diarrhoea was part of the clinical picture for only 14 per cent of the cases.
□ A mere six per cent of the patients had normal bowel habits.

The last point, of course, begs the question of what exactly is a so-called 'normal bowel habit'. Once again, there is no easy answer to that because there is such a great deal of variation from individual to individual. However, doctors tend to agree that 'normal' in this context means whatever has been the usual in the past for a given person when he or she was in good health, whether this meant as many as up to three bowel movements a day or as few as only one every three or four days and even fewer in some instances. Regularity in the pattern of bowel movements is considered much more telling than their frequency and therefore the pattern only falls outside the 'normal' when for one reason or another there is a major change over some period of time in the customary frequency.

Going back to what can be considered typical symptoms of IBS, the list of these can be formidable indeed and – apart from those already mentioned above – includes:

- Pain in the abdomen, particularly the kind of pain that is often described as an 'ache' rather than an actual pain.
- Excessive wind, which is often accompanied by a 'bloated' feeling. Also frequent belching or frequent flatulence, which may be accompanied by 'rumblings' in the abdomen.
- Occasional incontinence.
- Stools that can be described as 'pellet-like' or 'rabbit-like' or 'pebble-like' and even 'ribbon-shaped'.
- Frequent discomfort in the rectum, which may feel as though it is never fully emptied.
- Mucus in the stools; also the passing of mucus on its own or in between stools.
- A feeling of tightness around the waist.
- Experiencing difficulty or discomfort when bending down.

These are, however, but a few of the main symptoms that may be indicative of IBS. There are a lot more that are often associated with the disorder and these include:

- Poor appetite – which may result in weight loss.
- A frequent desire for food – which may result in weight gains.
- Backache.
- Headaches and/or migraines.
- Bouts of anxiety and/or depression, especially if these seem to happen most often shortly after having a meal.

□ In the case of women, periods that are painful and/or painful intercourse. Also a feeling that the IBS symptoms appear to get worse near the time when a period is due.

Apart from these, there are yet more symptoms that frequently seem to accompany IBS – that is people who suffer from IBS often have these symptoms, but they in themselves are not necessarily indicative of IBS. These include:

□ Trouble in and around the mouth which may manifest itself as soreness, a stinging of the tongue, a raw gullet or even swollen lips.

□ Difficulties in breathing; feelings of tightness in the chest.

□ A pulse that may be erratic – either sometimes too slow or too fast.

□ Sleep difficulties – trouble in dropping off, or waking in the middle of the night.

□ Feeling restless and/or loss of concentration.

□ Problems with fluid retention.

□ Having a hot flush shortly after eating.

□ Skin problems, in particular in the form of rashes.

□ Often feeling tired for no immediately obvious reason.

□ Waterworks problems, including cystitis that responds but little to antibiotics, and frequent urination.

□ Otherwise unexplained sweating, hot flushes and faintness.

□ Reduced sex drive.

As can be seen from the above, the one thing that is clear about the symptoms of IBS is that there is nothing clear-cut about them, covering as they do such a wide range of seemingly unconnected ailments, including some that just about everyone experiences now and then. To complicate the issue further, some of the symptoms listed, such as anxiety and depression, are difficult to quantify as to how severe they are, and may in many instances not be due to physical causes and may instead be the result of emotional or mental states.

What's more, the symptoms that may indicate IBS are quite often contradictory. For example, either a more voracious or a reduced appetite could be meaningful – and so too could be either weight loss or weight gain. So then how on earth can you begin to determine whether or not your symptoms are suggestive of IBS or may be due to completely different causes altogether?

Well, there are two answers to that question:

1) Firstly, you should never try to diagnose your symptoms yourself and you should always consult your doctor. There are many sound reasons for that: only a suitably qualified doctor is in a position to eliminate other diseases which may be giving rise to your problems; and, once a correct diagnosis has been made, only a doctor can prescribe the right treatment which takes into full account all other facts relating to your health in general; self-diagnosis can be a dangerous path to tread for all sorts of reasons, including the obvious ones that you may end up worrying needlessly over a disorder you haven't got or may treat yourself in quite the wrong way for the one you do have. So, and this is worth stressing, don't agonise too much about whether or not you're suffering from IBS. Leave it to your doctor to decide.

2) If you're someone who has occasional symptoms that suggest the possibility of IBS – but don't feel that these are either marked or frequent enough to warrant seeing your doctor – you may just want to find out what the chances are that it is indeed IBS that's troubling you. Well, the advice given above remains valid: you should still see your doctor, no matter how fleeting or minor your symptoms are, because if they're marked enough to cause you to be concerned about them, then they're meaningful enough to warrant a visit to your doctor. If, despite all that, you're still determined to avoid or postpone the best and most obvious way of finding out, read on and find out how doctors themselves decide whether a patient's problems are the result of IBS.

However, before doing that, there is something else you should bear in mind. You, as the sufferer, are only aware of the 'symptoms' of whatever it may be that you're suffering from. In medical terminology, symptoms are by definition those things which the patient complains about and which they usually bring to the attention of their doctor. When making an even simple and straightforward diagnosis, your doctor will of course take into account your symptoms, but he will also be guided by what 'signs' he may have observed during examination. There is quite a difference between the two which can be summed up as follows:

☐ **Symptom:** an indication of a disorder or disease noticed by the patient himself or herself. This becomes a 'presenting symptom' when it leads the patient to seek a doctor's advice.

☐ **Sign:** an indication of a specific disorder or disease that is observed by a doctor during examination but which is not apparent to the patient.

Quite often the signs may indeed be much more revealing than the symptoms, especially as so many symptoms may be indicative of a wide range of possible causes. This, of course, also means that any effort you may make at self-diagnosis will be based solely on symptoms because you can't possibly take into account any signs of which you're unaware. That's one more good reason why the diagnosis should be left to your doctor.

Let's go back to how doctors may reach a diagnosis of IBS. There are essentially two different approaches to this. The first one consists of eliminating by tests all other possible reasons for the problem and then, having found no structural or biochemical causes, and all the symptoms and signs being consistent with and characteristic of IBS, saying in effect: "Well, that is what it must be because it's certainly not anything else."

As you can imagine, although this is the approach that had been favoured by many professionals until recently, it is one that can be extremely time-consuming as investigation after investigation is carried out and test after test made, only to end up with negative findings. While there is some comfort for the patient in the fact that the findings turn out to be negative in the end, it can also involve a great deal of worry and stress before that happy conclusion is reached. What's more, that approach does place great demands upon an often already overstretched health service.

Aware that a diagnostic approach based upon negative findings had many failings, the medical profession has sought various ways of diagnosing IBS positively, that is on the pattern of symptoms instead of upon what investigations didn't reveal. Naturally enough, the wide scope and often contradictory variety of IBS symptoms made this a very difficult task indeed – for example, should the symptom of weight gain and/or loss be included in the criteria? And what about the various symptoms which could easily be the result of emotional problems – should they be taken into account? Many of these questions were never fully resolved, but an international working party of specialists did, over a period of time, come up with the following symptom criteria for IBS:

1) Abdominal pain that has some relationship to defecation and/or

2) A disturbance in the pattern of defecation, be this an alteration in timing, frequency or stool form, usually accompanied by . . .

3) Bloatedness or distension of the abdomen.

However, many experts felt that this description was much too condensed to be of real practical value in everyday practice. So other symptoms were added to this criteria to create what became known as the *Manning Criteria* – so named after the leader of the Bristol-based group of specialists who first used them in a paper published in the *British Medical Journal*. The Manning Criteria added the following six points to the three above:

4) The abdominal pains reduce in intensity after defecation.

5) The stools are looser when there is pain – or they have been looser ever since the pain became noticeable.

6) Defecation occurs more frequently when there is pain.

7) There is a frequent feeling of less than complete evacuation after defecation.

8) Passage of mucus occurs either frequently or occasionally through the rectum.

9) There is a frequent feeling of distension and/or bloating of the abdomen.

Although the nine points outlined above have been used widely both in clinical practice and epidemiological surveys, there were some that felt that there was a need to take into account three more points:

10) There is a frequent urgent need for defecation.

11) The stools are often runny or watery and this symptom alternates with stools that are solid.

12) There often is a need to strain to complete defecation.

Added together, these twelve symptoms are now accepted as pointers that indicate that there is intestinal dysfunction and very strongly suggest that the original cause of the pain lies somewhere in the colon. Additionally, these symptoms are especially suggestive of rectal irritability.

Of course, there is a need for several of the symptoms to be in existence to justify a diagnosis of IBS, and the greater the number of the symptoms presented, the greater the likelihood of IBS.

Summing up this 'positive' approach to diagnosing IBS, Dr K W Heaton, of the Bristol Royal Infirmary, concluded in *Towards Confident Management of Irritable Bowel Syndrome*: "Any of them (the symptoms above) can be caused by organic disease but the combination of several symptoms including rectal ones occurs in virtually no organic disease (except proctocolitis which is easy to diagnose). The vast majority of people with these symptoms have IBS."

It is, of course, possible for the layperson to use the same criteria to determine whether their symptoms are likely to be those of IBS. While the procedure seems simple enough, the previous warning about self-diagnosis still applies and diagnosis should remain a matter for your doctor. However, it can be interesting for a patient to see for themself just how closely their symptoms may match those that are considered to be typically indicative of the syndrome.

And just to clear up a point in the earlier quotation from Dr Heaton, 'proctocolitis' is an inflammation of the rectum and colon, the cause of which is usually ulcerative colitis. It is similar to 'proctitis' but in this instance only the rectum is affected by the inflammation and typical symptoms would include ineffectual straining to empty the bowels – a condition that is called 'tenesmus' – and is usually accompanied by bleeding. Both proctocolitis and proctitis are, as suggested, easily diagnosed by a doctor and you can rest assured that the existence of either would be quickly spotted in any routine examination.

The difficulty in confidently identifying IBS is that so many of the individual symptoms linked to it do occur for all sorts of other reasons and that therefore at the end of the day the doctor has to rely upon either eliminating all other possible sources of the symptoms or diagnose IBS positively on the basis of there being enough typical symptoms present. Despite all that, doctors do manage to diagnose IBS successfully although it must be added that in many cases this is not always necessarily through working their way through a check list as suggested above, but rather that cumulative clinical experience plays a big role as well. As one doctor said: "When I hear just the first few symptoms mentioned, I kind of get – if you'll pardon the pun – a gut feeling that tells me 'this is going to turn out to be IBS'. And I'm seldom wrong – although naturally enough I would never base a diagnosis on that alone and would always soldier on first through the whole diagnostic routine before reaching any conclusion."

A secondary difficulty in diagnosing IBS lies in the fact that so many people have some of the symptoms some of the time without, of course, actually having IBS itself. The prevalence of some of these symptoms was highlighted in a recent study in Bristol where a random sample of 1,038 women, aged between 25 and 69 years, and 858 men, aged between 40 and 69 years, were interviewed. The study showed the prevalence rates listed below – and, when reading these, please bear in mind that this was a random sample, that is of people in general, not of those who had complained of any particular symptoms or ailments previously.

☐ Complaining of recurrent abdominal pain – which is often described by the acronym 'RAP' with 'recurrent' being defined in this instance as more than six times in the previous year – which was often relieved by passing stools: 10.3 per cent of the women; 5.6 per cent of the men.

☐ Reporting experiences of 'RAP' linked with stools that were looser than usual: 6 per cent of the women; 3 per cent of the men.

☐ Reporting experiences of 'RAP' linked with stools that were passed more frequently than usual: 5 per cent of the women; 2.3 per cent of the men. It needs to be noted here that there was, of course, sizable overlap between the three different kinds of RAP with many of those interviewed having experienced two or all three at one time or another.

☐ Reporting frequent feelings of being bloated – 'frequent' in this context being defined as occurring at least one out of every four days: 15 per cent of the women; 6 per cent of the men.

☐ Feeling frequently that evacuation had been less than complete: 13 per cent of the women; 4.5 per cent of the men.

And so the list went on to cover all of the nine main IBS symptoms with each and every one of them being experienced frequently by a sizable proportion of the general population. But what was even more interesting was what emerged when these statistics were examined further to find out how many people had experienced more than just one symptom. The results of this were:

☐ Reporting that they had experienced any two – or more – of the nine main IBS symptoms: 24 per cent of the women; 11 per cent of the men.

☐ Reporting that they had experienced any three – or more – of the nine main IBS symptoms: 13 per cent of the women; 5 per cent of the men.

What was clear from this was that many of the symptoms of IBS occurred commonly all the time in people who didn't even feel they had a problem and who certainly wouldn't even consider there was a need to consult a doctor. Perhaps some of these people should have done so, because, once again to quote Dr Heaton: "… a quarter of the adult female population admitted to two or more symptoms. In other words they probably deserve the diagnosis of IBS."

Dr Heaton also pointed out that in his view even these figures were probably an underestimate because the study from which they had been derived had excluded women under the age of 25 years, who, he said, were the very people most likely to be prone to IBS. "Furthermore, the survey depended on people remembering their pains, discomfort and abnormal defecations, and on their being prepared to admit to them", he added. "In other words the survey excluded people who forgot their symptoms and symptom-deniers."

So, judging by the Bristol survey, the symptoms of IBS are so prevalent that it would be a rare person indeed who hasn't at least occasionally suffered one or more of them. How we react to these symptoms depends not only on their frequency and severity, but also upon our individual outlook. Some of us are natural 'pain tolerators' – that is, we can easily ignore and dismiss even comparatively severe discomfort if not actual pain. Others are 'pain-deniers' – people who can manage to ignore many symptoms by simply denying their existence to themselves. Most of us, of course, have a certain tolerance to pain and discomfort, but that only goes so far and when the symptoms reach what we consider to be an unacceptable stage, then seek help. But before anything can be done to alleviate IBS, it is vital that the underlying cause is established. That is by no means always an easy matter, as we shall discover in the next chapter.

Chapter 4

The Causes Of
Irritable Bowel Syndrome

A S WAS seen in the previous chapter, the symptoms of Irritable Bowel Syndrome are indeed many and extremely varied and it may therefore come as little surprise that there is an equally matching variety of theories as to why the disorder occurs in the first place.

There are, of course, many explanations as to why IBS may affect someone, but what is lacking is a clear-cut rationalisation to cover all aspects of the syndrome. This, once again, is not that surprising because there are many who believe that IBS is not one disorder but just a convenient catch-all label affixed to a number of quite separate ailments. This would also serve as a nice, logical reason why the symptoms can be so confusing and even self-contradictory.

That certainly is the view of one of Britain's top experts on the subject, Professor N W Read, of the Royal Hallamshire Hospital in Sheffield, who stated: "The many different presentations of this condition, the non-specific nature of many of the symptoms and the poor and variable response to treatment suggest that irritable bowel syndrome is no more than a convenient clinical category in which to place a large number of patients whose disease mechanisms are poorly understood. Therefore it seems likely that what we call Irritable Bowel Syndrome is not a single disease but consists of many different conditions."

He added that there was a historical precedent for that belief as what was now called IBS might in the past well have included other ailments – such as coeliac disease, colitis, lactose intolerance and bile acid deficiency – which can nowadays be identified as separate and specific entities.

So, if there are as it were many different forms of IBS, it would also follow that the causes – and, by implication, the treatments and/or cures – would also be manifold. That certainly seems to be the case because just about everything has at one time or another been blamed for being the cause of IBS. However, in the following exploration of potential causes, we will limit ourselves to those which have at least received a measure of medical endorsement at one time or another. The phrase 'at one time or another' is relevant because there seems to be a frequent shift in viewpoints on this subject and whatever causative factor it may be fashionable to blame IBS on today, may well be replaced by another one tomorrow.

Having said that, it remains a truism that the symptoms of IBS must have causes. After all, every physical problem has a physical reason as to why it happened – even though medical science may not as yet have unravelled the mechanisms at work. So it must be with IBS. However, the situation is made more complicated here because of the many different symptoms, each of which may have one or more potential causes. For example, take a very characteristic symptom like that of abdominal pain and it's pretty obvious that this could be the result of many different things, some of which are utterly unconnected with IBS as we understand it. And so it goes for most of the other symptoms with each and every one of them being capable of being explained away as the result of something other than IBS.

Someone once rather unkindly described IBS as 'a collection of symptoms looking for a disease'. While that might be a glib statement, there's just enough truth in it to warrant examining it further, as what makes IBS an entity is that it does consist of a collection of symptoms. When there is only one or perhaps two symptoms present, the diagnosis will hardly ever be that of IBS, but something much more specific. It is the very existence of what has also been called 'a collective of symptoms' that makes IBS as a whole much more than its individual parts.

Despite that, when looking for causes, we are forced once again to turn our attention to the symptoms in a piecemeal fashion, looking to see what might have provoked them in the first place.

WHAT IS KNOWN TO TRIGGER IBS

While there are many theories – some of them extremely conflicting – about the overall causes of IBS, there is one area where there is a great deal more of general agreement amongst the experts. This concerns what might be called 'trigger' points, or occurrences which preceded the first manifestations of the syndrome and to which its origins can often be traced back. Some of the more common trigger points include:

☐ A recent bout of gastro-enteritis which may have left the bowel in an over-sensitive state. Gastro-enteritis, of course, is just a name for what is colloquially known as 'holiday tummy' and in its broadest sense means an inflammation of the stomach or intestine. It is usually the result of an acute virus infection or bacteria or of food poisoning. Symptoms of the illness, which usually last three to five days or more, include vomiting and diarrhoea.

☐ The taking of antibiotics over a fairly long period of time as this can affect the natural bacteria in the body.

☐ A surgical operation that affected the abdominal or pelvic regions.

☐ Being physically run down for some time, whatever the cause of that might have been originally, such as recovering from another disease, or giving birth, or even having a condition that causes chronic physical pain.

☐ Being emotionally low – again the causes for this mental state are potentially many, but obvious examples include: marriage or relationship difficulties, work problems, bereavement, examinations and unemployment.

As can be seen from the above list, the sort of things that are implicated in possibly triggering off IBS fall into two major groups.

First of all, there are physical occurrences and secondly, there are the emotional and mental states, most of which are linked to stress in one fashion or another. For the time being, we will mainly ignore the role of stress which is covered fully in a later chapter, and concentrate instead on the physical causes.

Having identified some of the trigger mechanisms that are often responsible for bringing about the first symptoms of IBS, it is worth looking at the question of why some people are more likely to develop IBS than others or are already predisposed to it. After all, just about everyone will sooner or later experience gastro-enteritis, but not all of these will go on to develop IBS as a result.

These are just some of the things which experts believe can make someone a prime candidate for IBS:

☐ There may be some abnormality in the way the muscles of your gut propel its contents. This abnormality could be the result of genetic inheritance or it may have emerged following a gastro-intestinal infection. It has been found that many IBS sufferers have intestinal muscles that contract more strongly than usual and this can in turn cause spasm and pain.

☐ People's digestive tracts are not identical in their sensitivity and yours may just be one that is extra-sensitive and reacts more strongly than the average.

☐ The amount of mucus that is produced within the bowel also varies greatly and you may simply be someone who produces more of it than normal.

☐ Most of us can have mildly adverse reactions to various foods and in your case that may show up by your gut over-reacting to a food that 'doesn't agree with you'.

☐ You may have a condition known as 'incompetent sigmoid colon' which means that the performance of the last part of the colon is impaired to some degree, resulting in diarrhoea because not enough water will have been absorbed from the food residues before they are allowed to enter the rectum.

☐ As suggested earlier, you may be predisposed to IBS because for one reason or another – usually due to gastro-enteritis or taking antibiotics for a long time – there have been changes in the gut-dwelling useful bacteria that normally aid digestion and which no longer do their job as efficiently as before.

☐ You may have a tendency to hyperventilate – or over-breathe – and this has often been identified as leading to various gastro-intestinal problems because of swallowing air.

☐ You may have some problem with your blood sugar level which may be unstable. This can lead to poor nutrition which in turn may help precipitate a toxic colon.

☐ There may be a lack of certain essential vitamins in your diet, notably some of those in the B-complex, many of which are vital to the overall healthy functioning of the digestive system.

☐ Your production of digestive enzymes – those chemicals that break down the food to allow it to be absorbed into the body – may be impaired, perhaps as the result of a diet that is too high in refined foods.

☐ You may have too much Candida albicans – also known as 'thrush' – in your gut. This is a yeast which exists normally in the gut, but it can proliferate to harmful levels for a number of reasons, including the use of broad spectrum antibiotics as well as a diet that is too rich in sugar.

We'll be returning in greater detail to some of the points raised above in later chapters when we look at ways of treating IBS because, quite frequently, dealing with the triggering factor that made someone originally susceptible to the syndrome may at a later stage clear the symptoms.

MULTI-FACTORIAL CAUSES

Naturally enough it also follows that many of the factors outlined above may not just be predisposing but in many instances may be the actual cause and it can be difficult to draw a hard and fast line between the two. This distinction becomes even more blurred when you take into account the belief of many experts that the cause of IBS in a given case is often multi-factorial, meaning that it is due not to just one cause but to two or more factors interacting to cause the symptoms. For example, it may well be that someone does indeed have too much Candida albicans in their gut. However, although the yeast level is high, it doesn't cause any problems. Then, for one reason or another, a second predisposing factor – say, a high level of stress – comes into play as well and the two factors then combine to produce IBS symptoms. In this instance, it's also possible that the stress by itself – had it not been aided by the high proliferation of the Candida albicans – would not have been a sufficiently strong trigger to set off the IBS symptoms.

This multi-faceted aspect of causation does create many difficulties in both diagnosis and choice of treatment. While some possible causes – such as when Candida albicans is the culprit, or at least, as it were, a co-defendant – can be identified and quantified comparatively easily, others – such as mental stress levels – are not so simple to categorise. Many doctors, of course, won't agonise too much over this and will proceed to treat the more identifiable symptom and this may often bring results that are good enough so that there is no need for any further concern.

DISCOVERING THE CAUSE BY TREATING IT

Closely akin to the methodology above is identifying what may be the cause in a given instance by finding out what either cures or alleviates the symptoms. This may seem like putting the cart before the horse, but if, for example, good results are obtained by adding a bulking agent to the patient's diet, then it's a fairly simple matter to reach a kind of retrospective diagnosis which essentially says: "The cause must have been a lack of fibre and this has been proven because adding fibre to the diet got rid of the symptoms." It's perhaps not all that surprising that in the busy world of the general practitioner many patients are treated on that basis with often excellent results.

The degree and quality of response to treatment is not only a useful yardstick by which to establish original causes, but it is also perhaps the best way to categorise different kinds of IBS. In this way both the efficacy of treatments and the incidence rates of various types of IBS can be scientifically established and compared, which is vital if knowledge of the syndrome as a whole is to improve.

In a reference to 'response to treatment', Professor Read, who was quoted previously, stated: "In many respects this is the most reliable and useful criterion on which to sub-divide patients. The existing sub-sets of IBS such as lactose intolerance and bile acid diarrhoea have been established largely on the basis of effective response to treatment." But he added that there was little point in sub-dividing patients unless this led to sub-sets which could be treated in 'different, specific and effective' ways.

While the main likely causes and contributing factors to IBS have been outlined above, there are also other avenues currently under investigation and we will now look at these.

HORMONES

Many hormones are known to affect the gut with some of them creating additional movement within it and others inhibiting it. Add to this the fact that eating is what prompts the release of these hormones into the bloodstream and you can begin to understand why the idea of hormonal involvement in IBS has seemed so promising. Promising, yes, but the results of investigations into this direction have proven inconsistent. No conclusions have been drawn to date and the experts admit freely that a great deal more has to be learned about the hormones in the gut before even a tentative theory can be put forward.

MEDICATION

Many drugs that are used commonly in treating everyday ailments also have a potential to adversely affect gut functions. Included in the list of drugs that are now known to have side-effects on the gut are narcotics, beta-blockers, antacids and antibiotics. It is not unlikely that there may be many others which can also perhaps precipitate IBS-like symptoms in a particularly predisposed person.

FAT

This has been clearly identified as a trigger in some cases of IBS with the mechanism at work appearing to be that the fatty acids in the fat stimulate the release of *cholecystokinin* – a hormone that is secreted by the cells of the duodenum when it is occupied by partly digested food. The cholecystokinin makes the gall-bladder contract and thereby expel bile into the intestine as well. It also stimulates the production of digestive enzymes by the pancreas. These actions lead to increased colonic motor activity which, in turn, could create IBS symptoms.

Although this chapter is concerned with the causes of IBS, there are three items which also need to be mentioned briefly at this time – we will return to these in greater detail in later chapters – and these are dietary fibre, diet in general and lactose intolerance, all three of which have a profound effect upon how our digestive system works. The big question, of course, is whether these are truly causes of IBS or merely factors which further adversely affect a digestive system which is already IBS-prone. While making changes in diet – including making it milk-free or increasing the amount of fibre – has been found to 'cure' countless IBS sufferers, it by no means follows that the 'wrong' food, milk products or lack of fibre were the original cause of the syndrome. In this context it is worthwhile to recall what was said earlier about the causation of IBS being almost certainly multi-factorial in most instances. If that is so, then diet deficiencies can only be part of the reason why the symptoms arose in the first place.

In some ways, of course, the question of whether diet is a true cause of IBS remains one that is only of academic interest as far as most sufferers are concerned. Quite understandably, patients – and many doctors, for that matter – take a very pragmatic view: if adding or deleting something to one's diet gets rid of the symptoms, then whatever was lacking or in the diet originally must have been the cause of the trouble. However, for the purpose of this book, the diet-related aspects of IBS will be covered separately in the relevant chapters which follow.

As far as discovering the causes – and just about everyone agrees that there are no doubt several of these – is concerned, it seems that we will have to wait some time before these become fully known. In the meantime, it is reassuring to know that although modern medicine may be still somewhat in the dark about what makes IBS appear, it does offer lots of extremely efficient ways of treating the symptoms, and that is what really matters as far as most of us are concerned.

The first step, of course, towards benefiting from these treatments, is to consult your doctor and that's what the next chapter is all about.

Chapter 5

How Your Doctor Can Help You

A S YOU'LL have read in the previous chapter, there are indeed many good reasons why you should consult your doctor if you're suffering from symptoms that are indicative of Irritable Bowel Syndrome. Nevertheless, it is appreciated that although sufferers may theoretically accept these reasons, they will still often be reluctant to make an appointment.

This reluctance to seek help from the one single source that is most able to provide it usually stems from one or more of the following reasons:

- ☐ So many of the symptoms of IBS are of such a personal nature that patients can find it difficult to bring themselves to discuss them openly with someone else.
- ☐ Some people will postpone or avoid consulting their doctor because they fear that the diagnosis will be bad. To put it bluntly, just about everyone who has experienced recurrent bowel problems over a period of time must wonder whether these could just possibly be due to cancer. Almost invariably, this is not the case, but the thought that it just might be does put people off from finding out what they think might be the worst.
- ☐ By seeking medical help, you're acknowledging that your problems are of more than just a temporary nature and therefore unlikely to disappear of their own accord.
- ☐ You may have heard stories of how people with symptoms that sounded similar to yours were placed by their doctors on diets that

were so unpleasant or restrictive that their lives became miseries.

☐ You may think that your symptoms are not severe enough to warrant you 'troubling' your doctor by taking up their time unnecessarily. After all, they are busy and there are people out there who are really sick and need your doctor's time more than you do.

☐ You've arrived at the conclusion – perhaps quite correctly – that you're suffering from IBS and you've been told or read that it can be very difficult to treat and the success rate for treatment is not all too good.

☐ You fear that your doctor may just tell you that 'it's all in your mind'. In fact, you yourself may have managed to convince yourself that this is the case and if that is so, what can they do to help you?

☐ You think that the discomfort or pains you suffer are part and parcel of your particular lifestyle and are just something you have to accept as best you can. Or you fear that you will be told that you'll have to change your habits in a way that you're not prepared to do, such as, for example, having to give up smoking.

These – and doubtlessly many other variations upon the same basic themes – are the main reasons why IBS sufferers may keep on postponing seeking help. It is a great shame that this should happen, because each and every one of these reasons (or to be blunt once again, excuses) doesn't hold up if you care to examine them more logically and less emotionally.

Let's look at them one by one:

The reluctance to discuss personal details relating to bowel habits. This is, of course, perfectly understandable as this is certainly not a suitable subject for general conversation. However, the consultation with your doctor is rather different because they will without doubt have encountered this situation many, many times before and will also be experienced in putting you at your ease while you discuss the specifics of your problems. There's no need to worry too much about which words to use, as long as their meaning is clear.

Incidentally, words like 'faeces', 'stools', 'bowel motions' are perfectly acceptable and indeed are found in all the best dictionaries. Once you've broached the subject, you will certainly find that both the interview and examination phases of the consultation proceed smoothly with your doctor taking the lead by asking you the relevant questions.

Postponing seeing your doctor because you fear that the news will be bad. This is, of course, a perfectly understandable reaction, but is nevertheless one that doesn't serve your own interests best. First of all, the odds are very, very strongly in your favour that your doctor's examination will only reveal symptoms of IBS – and that reassurance in itself should take a great worry off your mind. Secondly, in the rare instances – and it must be stressed that these are rare indeed – when there is suspicion or evidence that something more sinister than IBS is responsible for the symptoms, then it's clearly to your advantage to have any other disease diagnosed as soon as possible: the chances of successful treatment increase dramatically in ratio to early discovery. Logic in fact suggests that the more you have reason to fear that something nastier than IBS may be involved, the more you owe it to yourself to seek the correct advice as soon as possible; by doing so, you will give yourself the best chance of overcoming whatever it might be.

The unwillingness to accept that your symptoms are going to remain with you unless you have something done about them. This, once again, is a perfectly natural reaction. Most of us will play a waiting game for a while in the hope that whatever might be ailing us will go away of its own accord. But – and this is a big but – you musn't overdo this. If your symptoms are persistent or recurrent and if they are severe enough to cause you to be concerned about them, then you owe it to yourself to seek advice even if just for the sake of your own peace of mind.

You're put off from seeing your doctor because of stories you've heard from other people. Yes, this probably happens to all of us at one time or another. We think we have a specific problem, mention it casually to a friend or acquaintance who then proceeds to tell us a horrific tale of someone who had 'the very same thing'. First of all, the chances are that the story will have become embellished in the telling; secondly, although your friend may say it was 'the same thing', that is not all that likely to be truly the case. Many, many different diseases may present themselves with remarkably similar symptoms, but the underlying causes – and therefore the treatments available and their rates of success – will vary tremendously. Even if IBS was specifically diagnosed in the case you're being told about, it certainly doesn't mean that your treatment will follow the same course. As has been seen in the previous chapter, IBS can stem from a wide variety of causes. What's more, the symptoms by themselves certainly don't always identify the causes in a particular case. For example, just because your gastric pain is in the same place of the abdomen as someone else's doesn't mean that the reasons for it are the same or that the treatments for it will be identical. Second-hand or even third-hand stories about how a very restrictive diet made someone's life a misery are hardly worth listening to as there is no reason to believe that even if the treatment for your specific symptoms were to include a diet plan that it would be the same one.

You don't want to 'trouble' your doctor with a 'minor' problem. If the problem is severe enough to cause you to think about it, then it's also severe enough to warrant you getting expert advice for it. Any doctor will tell you that pain or discomfort which occurs frequently needs investigation, if only to ensure that it is not potentially dangerous to your overall health. As far as taking up your doctor's time, as long as your worries over your problems are causing you genuine concern, you're just as entitled to your share of their time as any other patient.

Not seeking help because you know that IBS can be difficult to treat. Yes, it's true that a few forms of IBS can be difficult to treat, mainly because it can be hard to identify the cause of the symptoms. Many more types of IBS do, however, respond extremely well and rapidly to comparatively simple measures, and the chances are that this will be so in your case. Even were it otherwise, surely it's better to get treatment than just to keep suffering the symptoms.

You think your doctor is going to say that it's all in your mind. Well, that could just happen, but not quite in that form as your doctor may come to the conclusion that your pains originate from stress and that the best way to treat you is to deal with the sources of the stress and thereby overcome the IBS symptoms that way. Even so, your doctor is hardly likely to say 'it's all in your mind', but instead will offer you help and, if need be, treatment to reduce your stress levels.

You believe that your symptoms are just something that you have to accept. You should never be prepared to live with pain or recurrent discomfort until you've at least explored what can be done about it. It's true that in certain instances the successful treatment of IBS may make demands upon you and you may have to alter some lifetime habits. If you'd sooner stick to your old ways and suffer the pain, that choice always remains open to you. But you do owe it to yourself to first find out what can be done and most of the treatments – unfortunately not all – make very little if any demand upon the patient.

So there are really no good or logical reasons to keep on postponing consulting your doctor – and plenty of good ones why you should do so just as soon as reasonably convenient! Remember, the sooner you see your doctor, the sooner you will learn what exactly is the matter with you, and the sooner you will be getting treatment which will make you feel better. What's more, you'll no longer have to worry about whether or not to seek medical advice!

Having made an appointment with your doctor, there are a few simple and practical things you can do in preparation for your visit which may help them reach a diagnosis more easily. These include:

□ Making a reasonably detailed list of your bowel habits. This should include frequency of defecation (once a day, twice a day, every three days, or whatever); whether the frequency is broadly speaking regular, that is occurring at more or less the same time of day or whether the intervals vary greatly; whether the stools are usually firm, solid, runny, pellet-like, and whether their consistency is more or less the same all the time or very changeable.

☐ Other questions that you may be asked about your bowel habits might include: Do you experience pain or discomfort when using the toilet? Is there evidence of mucus? Has there ever been any evidence of bleeding? Do you often feel that evacuation of the rectum is only partial? Do you have to strain a great deal to pass bowel motions? Does this also cause any pain or discomfort elsewhere? Do the various pains ease after you've been to the toilet? Think about your answers to these questions in advance.

☐ You should also jot down as clearly as you can remember when pain or discomfort which you think is linked with IBS strikes you. Is the pain there most of the time or only now and then? Does it seem to occur at a particular time of day? Does it seem to occur at a more or less set interval after you've had a meal – or eaten a particular kind of food? Is the pain usually in the same part of the abdomen? Does the pain seem to travel about around the abdomen? Do you suffer from wind (flatulence) or burping?

Of course, your answers to most of these questions will almost automatically raise supplementary ones: "How long has this – the pain, the discomfort, whatever – been going on? Can you remember when you first started to notice this? Has the pattern or severity since then remained more or less the same or has it recently changed in any major way?"

Naturally enough, it's also very worthwhile to make a note if you yourself have been able to link the manifestation of any symptom to any specific event or occurrence. For example, if you've found that your digestion reacts badly after you've eaten Chinese food or drunk red wine, that information may be extremely useful to your doctor. It's also worthwhile spending a few moments thinking back to particularly bad bouts of IBS and seeing whether you can identify a possible cause for it. The converse is also true; if certain foods or certain activities – this could include going for a walk, or having a nap, or doing a few breathing exercises – reduce your symptoms, that too may be indicative of the nature of your IBS. Summing this up, jot down on a notepad anything that you yourself have discovered which brings on your symptoms or makes them more severe or lessens them.

There is another list you might care to make in preparation for your appointment and this is one of various questions to which you'd like the answers. Your doctor may, in fact, automatically cover all of these points as your examination proceeds, but it's just as well to be prepared beforehand.

Such a list could include questions like:

□ **What is it exactly that I'm suffering from?** Knowing the exact name of the diagnosed ailment will make it easier for you to – if you wish – look up more details about it in medical reference books like this one.

□ **What is the cause of my problems?** If the diagnosis is one of IBS, your doctor may be hard put to answer this one because as we have seen previously, the causes are often extremely difficult to ascertain with any degree of certainty. They may well, however, be able to offer you an educated guess as to why you in particular have certain specific symptoms. If your ailment is diagnosed as something other than IBS, then this question may well be of great importance as the cause may be one about which you can do something.

□ **Can my illness go on to affect other parts of my body?** Is it likely to get much worse – or better – of its own accord?

□ **Could I possibly have something else – that is another problem altogether but one which causes similar symptoms to appear?** Naturally, you'll have to be very diplomatic in raising this issue as no doctor likes having their diagnosis questioned, but some will at times freely admit that while they believe their diagnosis to be the right one, it just could be that your problems stem from something else. If that's the case, that could be useful information for you because it may enable you to think of other relevant symptoms which may cause a revision of the diagnosis.

☐ **What's the best treatment in my case?** Doctors, for very good reasons, tend to operate on the principle that in the first instance the best treatment is the mildest of those indicated. If that brings satisfactory results, all's well and good; if the results are less than adequate, they will then proceed with a more energetic therapy. 'Best' in this connection is a relative term, meaning what is best in view of the known circumstances.

☐ **For how long and how often will I need to continue with the treatment? How long will it be before I can reasonably expect an improvement in my condition?** This information is very important because many medications may require quite a length of time before they start benefiting you and it's not unknown for a patient to give up on a course of medication much too soon because 'it's not making any difference'. The treatment might well have solved the problem if the patient had persevered with it long enough to give it a chance to work. Knowing beforehand how long it may take to see results will make it all the more likely that you will comply with the treatment for the time it needs.

☐ **Are there possible side-effects of which I should be aware?** In many ways this can be a tricky one for your doctor to answer. Just about every kind of medication has some known associated side-effects. That doesn't mean that everyone who takes that particular prescription also experiences the side-effects, just that it's possible, if not necessarily likely, that this may happen. Doctors are also aware of the fact that when patients know what side-effects may occur, they can lead themselves into believing that they're experiencing them. So there's a fine line to be drawn here between giving too much information or too little.

☐ **Can this treatment interact unfavourably with any medication which I'm taking currently for other problems?** Your doctor will, of course, be aware of what prescribed drugs you're using, but many preparations that can be bought without a prescription at any chemist's can also cause interactions. If you're regularly using any 'over-the-counter' medications, it's a good idea to tell your doctor what these are.

Naturally, it will probably not be necessary for you to ask all of these questions as the answers to many of them may well become obvious as your examination progresses. But, it's generally better to ask too many questions than too few. In this context it's worth quoting what Dr Cynthia Carver, a noted expert on doctor-patient relationships and a government medical officer, had to say: "Learn as much as possible about your disease or problem. Doctors can make mistakes and your best defence against this possibility is knowledge. The key to receiving careful medical treatment lies in being a well-informed consumer."

Normally, your consultation with your doctor will consist of several well-defined phascs:

1) They will hear your account of the various symptoms that made you come and see them.

2) You'll be asked a number of questions to clarify or amplify your description of the symptoms.

3) You may be asked some additional questions before your doctor proceeds to the examination phase.

4) Your doctor may proceed with a number of tests to look for signs. One of these will almost certainly be a rectal examination – see the next chapter for fuller details about this and other tests and investigations.

5) Upon completing their examination, your doctor may have a few supplementary questions to put to you. They will then either offer their diagnosis or suggest that it may be necessary to carry out a few more tests which may require your attendance at an out-patients' clinic at your local hospital.

6) In most cases, however, this won't be necessary and your doctor will suggest a course of treatment to deal with the symptoms. What this treatment consists of will, of

course, depend upon the nature of your IBS symptoms and the various approaches to this are described fully in later chapters of this book.

This brings your consultation to the stage where you have your opportunity to raise any points which may not already have been answered. Don't be afraid to ask questions as most doctors will agree with the general proposition that a well-informed patient is one who is also more likely to be motivated strongly enough to comply fully – that is follow instructions – with the requirements of the treatment. As the best treatment in the world won't achieve results if the patient doesn't adhere to it, doctors appreciate that supplying necessary information can be an extremely important part of the therapy as a whole.

Chapter 6

Tests And Investigations

WHILE THERE are a great many different kinds of tests available to determine whether various parts of the digestive system are functioning correctly, there unfortunately simply isn't one that will specifically reveal Irritable Bowel Syndrome as such.

This means that, depending upon the severity of the symptoms and the age of the patient, various investigations are often carried out with each and every one of them revealing only that all is well. Of course, these findings are still extremely important because they at least allow the doctor to exclude other possible causes for the symptoms. One of the difficulties in diagnosing IBS lies in the fact that many of its characteristic symptoms can be equally typical of a wide range of other digestive disorders, such as inflammatory bowel disease, bacterial infections, diverticular disease, parasitic infections and certain tumours. If there is the slightest possibility that one of these may be responsible for your symptoms, your doctor will want to ascertain whether or not they are implicated.

When dealing with what they suspect will probably turn out to be IBS, doctors are well aware of the fact that most tests and investigations will merely confirm what they thought to be the case all along. Nevertheless – and despite the current trend to seek to diagnose IBS on a positive rather than a negative basis – your doctor may well think it wise to ensure that their initial diagnosis is correct by asking for various investigations, although they will almost certainly expect that the results of these will merely allow them to exclude other causes.

This, of course, means that you shouldn't become unduly worried if you're asked to attend a hospital clinic for additional investigations. This should not be taken as an indication that your doctor believes that there's something seriously amiss, but rather that he is making doubly certain that there isn't.

During your initial examination, your doctor will probably do the following simple tests:

☐ Look carefully at your abdomen for any signs of irregularity or unusual distension.

☐ Touch and prod the abdomen to find out if there are any signs of either tenderness or rigidity.

☐ Carry out a rectal examination.

This last one sounds more daunting than it is in fact and really is nothing to be worried out. Usually, you will be asked to undress below the waist, lie down on the examination couch and assume a position in which you're on your left side while bending both of your legs slightly upwards. Having first put on a pair of thin rubber gloves, your doctor will then gently and slowly insert a finger into the rectum, moving it slightly about inside so that he can feel the inner surface. Although this procedure may be somewhat embarrassing for the patient, rest assured that it is certainly not painful and at worst just slightly uncomfortable. As far as the embarrassment is concerned, try to put this out of your mind while remembering that this kind of examination is a routine one for your doctor who will no doubt do their best to put you at your ease.

BLOOD TESTS

This is another likely test because it can reveal, amongst many other things, evidence of generalised infection, anaemia, and also provide information about how well your liver and kidneys are functioning.

In most instances, the required blood sample will be taken by your doctor during your visit. The procedure is straightforward: to begin, an alcohol swab is used to clean a small area of your skin, usually on the upper arm; then a fine needle attached to a syringe is inserted into a vein and a small amount of blood drawn into the syringe by suction.

STOOL SPECIMEN

Your doctor may think it worthwhile to ask you to supply a stool specimen so that it can be sent to the laboratory for examination. This is usually done for two reasons: firstly, to see if there are minimal specks of blood in it, specks that could be so small as to be completely undetectable by the naked eye; and, secondly, to find out if there are any unusual bacteria present.

It may take a few days before your doctor gets the results of these tests and you will therefore be asked to make another appointment to see your doctor a week or so later. At that time, they will either be satisfied that there is nothing organically wrong with you or – if they have the slightest doubt – will refer you to a hospital gastroen-terologist for further investigation. Once again, it's worth stressing that the mere fact of being referred should not cause you undue worry. In most instances, it's simply a case of 'better safe than sorry' as the hospital has facilities for carrying out investigations that are beyond the scope of a general practitioner.

While there is a large battery of possible tests and investigations, the following are the most likely ones.

SIGMOIDOSCOPY

This is a procedure that allows the specialist actually to look inside the rectum and the lower colon by using an instrument called a 'sigmoidoscope', which in its most common form is a tube about 25 centimetres (about ten inches) long with some sort of illumination at the end of it. There are also flexible sigmoidoscopes which use fibre optic technology and can be as long as 60 centimetres (about two feet) and even more.

During this examination, you will be asked to lie in more or less the same position as that used for a rectal examination. Although no one would claim that sigmoidoscopy was a comfortable procedure for the patient, neither is it usually painful in any way. Uncomfortable, certainly; painful, no. Despite that, if you should at any time during the examination feel any pain, you should tell the doctor so immediately. There can, however, be one curious side-effect of the examination and this happens because the sigmoidoscope has a small air pump built into it and the doctor may use this to partially inflate the bowel so as to improve both access and the view. Not uncommonly, some of the air pumped into the bowel remains trapped there and gives rise to bloatedness, wind and flatulence some time later.

The purpose of sigmoidoscopy, of course, is to check for signs of abnormality of any kind, such as inflammation or the presence of any growths, whether these be non-cancerous or cancerous.

In most instances, sigmoidoscopy will reveal nothing out of the ordinary. Negative though this finding may be, it is nevertheless usually of great comfort to the patient who thereby learns that certain possibilities are no longer to be feared. Incidentally, there are two small findings which may result and which by themselves are quite indicative that IBS is indeed the problem.

The first of these may happen when the doctor introduces the sigmoidoscope and sees quite strong and frequent contractions of the lower end of the bowel. This occurrence – known as the 'winking sign' – is frequently associated with the type of IBS that is marked by constipation and abdominal pain.

The second thing that may happen is that the sigmoidoscope – particularly when the bellows are used to slightly inflate the colon – may trigger off the very exact discomfort that the patient had been complaining about. Although setting off the discomfort may not be all that welcome to the patient, this is in fact to be regarded as a good sign because it usually indicates that the source of the pain lies in the muscular actions of the bowel wall instead of something which might be more difficult to deal with.

BARIUM ENEMA

Barium sulphate is a salt that is insoluble in water and therefore when taken internally remains opaque to X-rays. As such it provides an extremely useful contrast medium for the radiography of the intestines and the stomach.

The usual procedure for barium enemas requires the patient to have nothing or very little to eat the night before, and to take a laxative to ensure that they open their bowels on the day.

In the hospital's radiology department, a tube will be inserted into the rectum to allow the entry of a small quantity of the barium, which looks like thickish white liquid. To allow the barium to flow into the various parts of the gut, the patient will be asked to lie down on a table which can be tilted in various ways so that gravity plays its part in distributing the barium. A number of X-rays are then taken from various angles and after these have been processed, the barium will show up clearly on the plates allowing the doctor to see any irregularities in the gut.

In some instances, normal X-rays may be taken before and/or after those with the barium for comparison purposes. At the end of the procedure, the barium fluid will either be extracted from the colon or eliminated as a somewhat runny bowel movement.

Once again, this investigation is uncomfortable rather than painful, although not uncommonly it is followed by a moderately severe attack of wind which subsides of its own accord in due course.

LACTOSE INTOLERANCE

Lactose is a very special kind of sugar, consisting of one molecule of glucose and one of galactose, which is only found in milk. In a normal digestive system, the lactose is split into its two constituent sugars by the action of the enzyme lactase which, as you may recall from the previous chapter on the digestive system, is secreted in the small intestine. This enzyme can, however, be missing or be of low activity in some people, in particular those of certain Eastern or

African races, and this inability to absorb lactose properly is known as lactose intolerance.

There is a fairly simple way of establishing whether someone may be suffering from lactose intolerance. It is known as the *hydrogen breath test*, which you'll be pleased to know involves nothing more unpleasant than fasting overnight and the next morning drinking a specific quantity of lactose and having samples taken of your breath at hourly intervals for the next three hours.

How the test works is quite straightforward. If you don't have the enzyme to digest the lactose either in a strong enough form or in sufficient quantity, the lactose will not be absorbed as it would have been otherwise in the small intestine and will instead travel on to the large intestine. There resident bacteria in the gut will break it down and during this process generate hydrogen which – via the blood-stream – will eventually reach your lungs. As you breathe out, the quantity of hydrogen in your exhaled breath will reveal whether you have lactose intolerance.

The above are the three main tests which may be used to eliminate other causes in instances of suspected IBS. If none of these investigations reveal anything amiss, then your doctor or specialist will almost certainly settle for a diagnosis of IBS.

The extent to which various other tests and investigations should be used to exclude the possibility of organic disease when IBS is the main suspect can be a matter for wide-ranging discussion – and disagreement – amongst the specialists.

Here is what one leading expert, Dr P A Cann, of the Middles-brough General Hospital, had to say on the subject:

"My normal practice is to have a full blood count, plasma viscosity check and a sigmoidoscopic investigation, the latter partly because it has a therapeutic reassuring effect." Dr Cann, however, added that if the patient were aged over 40 years or if there was a recent history of significant weight loss, then further investigations would also be undertaken. And in instances where diarrhoea was one of the major presenting symptoms, a biopsy would be taken as well as a stool culture done.

Although the extent of investigations is a matter for the individual doctor or specialist, Dr Cann did point out that such testing did not always reveal a great deal. For example, there was a study of 84 patients with suspected IBS who each were put through a whole gamut of tests – many, many more than usual – and these included:

- Full blood count and ESR.
- Plasma urea/electrolytes/calcium levels.
- Liver function testing.
- Rectal biopsy.
- Stool microscopy and stool culture.
- Barium meal and follow through.
- Barium enema.
- Testing of thyroid function.
- Faecal fat excretion.
- Serum folate and vitamin B12 levels.
- Schilling test – this assesses the patient's capacity to absorb vitamin B12 from the bowel. The procedure consists of giving radioactive vitamin B12 by mouth and collecting the urine over a 24-hour period, during which a normal patient will excrete at least 10 per cent of the original dose.
- 14C-Glycocholate breath test which can determine the levels of bile function.
- Lactose tolerance test.
- Urinary 5-hydroxy-indole acetic acid test.

Now you might have thought that such an intensive investigation of just about all possible aspects of the digestive system would have yielded a great deal of information about the 84 patients involved. Not so, according to Dr Cann, who stated: "In only two patients (out of the 84) was a relevant alternative diagnosis found – one was a coeliac and one had giardiasis." Coeliac disease is a condition in which the small intestine fails to digest and absorb food properly and is thought to affect somewhat more than one per cent of the population in general. The cause of the disorder is due to the sensitivity of the intestinal lining to the protein gliadin, which is found in the gluten in the germ of wheat and rye, and this causes atrophy of both the digestive and absorptive cells of the gut. Giardiasis – also known as 'Lambliasis' – is caused by the presence of the parasitic prozoan 'Giardia lamblia' in the small intestine. Infection is usually the result of eating food contaminated with cysts containing the parasite. If present in large numbers, the parasites can interfere with the absorption of food through the gut wall. Symptoms include many very similar to those of IBS and the disease normally responds well to oral doses of either quinacrine or metronidazole.

The study mentioned above is by no means unique and there have been several others which sought to pinpoint just how worthwhile extensive testing and investigations really are when a patient presents all the characteristics of IBS without any additional signs that could indicate some other disease. Broadly speaking, all of these surveys came to a similar conclusion: there seldom is much to be learned from additional testing and that therefore it is sensible to limit the extent of this. This limitation, of course, not only saves hospital time and money, but equally importantly, may save a great deal of stress on the part of the patient who otherwise would be sent on a seemingly endless round of test after test, all of which would be unlikely to produce anything of substance to contribute to the diagnosis.

Although doctors nowadays broadly agree that there is generally little point in pursuing investigation after investigation, there is one very important exception to this which arises in the case of patients who are into middle age – this meaning those either over 40 or 45 years of age, depending upon who you ask. These patients, who because of their age automatically are at higher risk of possible tumours than younger ones, should usually have a colonoscopy. This is a procedure essentially similar to a sigmoidscopy but which allows a larger part of the colon to be viewed by using a 'colonoscope' which also makes it possible, if needed, to remove, using flexible forceps, small specimens from the gut for later microscopic examination. This instrument can also be used to remove *polyps* – which are growths, usually benign – that can occur on the wall of the bowel. The technique used for this varies according to the size and location of the polyp, but it is usually done by cutting across the base of the polyp with a 'snare', that is a sharp wire loop, through which is passed a high-frequency diathermy current to coagulate the blood. Polyps in the bowel can, of course, give rise to some of the symptoms associated with IBS, in particular blood-marked faeces.

Apart from the exception noted above, it's quite clear that in the vast majority of IBS cases there is little to be gained from extensive investigations and testing. Should the IBS be attributable to stress, this may even make its symptoms worse as the patient worries about what each and every test may reveal.

Summing up, it can be safely said that, once all the tests that seemed indicated have been carried out, in the vast majority of cases the doctor or specialist will usually be left to consider two facts:

1) The symptoms are not due to any determinable organic cause.

2) They are broadly speaking within the range of IBS.

On that basis, the diagnosis of IBS will almost certainly be made and the next step will be to consider how best to treat it. Just as there is a bewildering variety of potential causes and reasons why someone may be predisposed to IBS, there is an equally vast choice in potential treatments either to cure it or relieve its symptoms. In the next chapter, we will take an initial look at the many different approaches to treatment which are available.

Chapter 7

Treatments For
Irritable Bowel Syndrome

I T'S NOT surprising that an ailment such as Irritable Bowel
Syndrome – which can present itself through a wide and even
contradictory range of symptoms – has a wide variety of different
treatments linked to it.

Although each type of treatment will be examined in greater detail
later, let us first of all look at the main categories:

☐ Medications that are prescribed by your doctor. These can include
  bulking agents as well as other laxatives, depending upon the
  nature of the symptoms.

☐ Another type of frequently prescribed treatment is that which uses
  anti-spasmodic drugs, whose function it is to reduce spasm in the
  colon.

☐ Your doctor may also prescribe tranquillisers or antidepressants
  in certain instances if they feel that your IBS symptoms are the
  result of mental stress.

☐ Linked to the above is the possibility of using psychotherapeutic
  techniques as well as possibly hypnotherapy.

☐ Then there are meditation, relaxation and other techniques all of
  which aim at promoting physical well-being by relaxing the mind.

☐ There are also many different kinds of so-called 'alternative
  therapies', ranging from herbalism to aromatherapy.

☐ Last, but by no means least, as in fact many people believe that
  this represents the single most important approach to treating IBS,
  is the question of diet.

In this chapter, we shall concentrate on the three main forms of 'medical' treatment, that is bulking agents, laxatives and antispasmodics, and return to the other treatments later.

BULKING AGENTS

These work to relieve constipation by increasing the faecal mass and this in turn stimulates peristalsis, the wave-like movements that propel the contents of the gut along its length. There are many different bulk-forming drugs and all should be approached with a degree of caution as too much of a good thing can indeed be harmful. It is also extremely important that an adequate liquid intake is maintained to avoid the possibility of intestinal obstruction. Patients who take preparations that swell when brought into contact with a liquid should be counselled that these should always be carefully swallowed with water and should not be taken shortly before retiring for the night.

Some of the main bulk-forming drugs are:

BRAN. Unprocessed wheat – or oat – bran, usually taken with either other food or fruit juice, is considered to be a most effective bulk-former for many people. There are, however, some patients who don't tolerate bran very well and then other bulk-forming drugs have to be used instead. Another way of taking in bran is in a finely ground form as in bran bread or biscuits.

Some of the more commonly prescribed bran-based medications include: *Fybranta tablets* (manufacturers, Norgine) and *Proctofibe tablets* (Roussel).

ISPAGHULA HUSK. This is obtained from the seed husks of the plantain 'Plantago ovata' and is a rich source of so-called 'dietary fibre'. Dietary fibre is defined as that part of a plant which cannot be digested by enzymes or acid in the human gastrointestinal tract, although some of the fibre is broken down by the bacteria which colonise the large bowel. Ispaghula husk is made of both water soluble and water insoluble dietary fibre and these link to form a

63

matrix that can absorb up to 30 to 40 times its own weight in water.

The husk helps relieve constipation by passing in an undigested form down the gastrointestinal tract to the colon where the presence of the hydrated fibre mass causes the natural stimulation of peristalsis, which then leads to the passing of bulky and soft stools. One other benefit of the husk is that its fibre mass helps support the growth of natural colonic bacteria which increases the stool bulk.

Some possible side-effects are associated with Ispaghula husk and these include: abdominal distension, usually in a mild form; and flatulence, which normally resolves fairly quickly of its own accord.

The use of the husk is contra-indicated where there is intestinal obstruction, or faecal impaction, or colonic atony (this being a state in which the muscles of the bowel are floppy and lack their normal elasticity), such as might be found in senile megacolon, a condition that is marked by the dilatation – and also possible lengthening – of the colon. Megacolon is usually the result of long-standing constipation, or of ulcerative colitis, or of Hirschsprung's disease, a congenital condition in which the rectum and possibly part of the lower colon have failed to develop a normal nerve network. This last condition, however, usually becomes apparent in the first few weeks of life when it is treated by surgery.

Some of the more commonly prescribed husk-based formulations include: *Fybogel granules*, effervescent (manufacturers: Reckitt & Colman); *Isogel granules* (A & H); *Metamucil powder* (Procter and Gamble); and *Regulan powder*, effervescent (Procter and Gamble).

METHYLCELLULOSE. This is an alternative to Ispaghula husk with similar water-absorbing properties and the contra-indications and possible side-effects are the same.

Commonly prescribed preparations include: *Methylcellulose mixture* and *Celevac* (manufacturers: Monmouth).

STERCULIA. This is another bulk-former with the same contra-indications and possible side-effects as those listed above.

Commonly prescribed preparations include: *Normacol granules*, formerly known as Normacol Special (manufacturers: Norgine); and

Normacol Plus granules, formerly known as Normacol Standard (Norgine).

OTHER LAXATIVES

While constipation is often one of the symptoms of IBS, the approach to dealing with this will generally be through either making appropriate changes in the diet or incorporating one of the bulk-formers described above in it. Seldom will stimulant laxatives be used because their effect can often be too harsh and in any case will not help 're-educate' the bowel.

Nevertheless, it seemed right to include a brief description of some of the more commonly used laxatives.

STIMULANT LAXATIVES – The better known of these are usually based upon either *bisacodyl* or members of the *anthraquinone group*, such as senna. They do increase intestinal motility, but may often cause abdominal cramp. They are contra-indicated if there is a possibility of intestinal obstruction and prolonged use can precipitate the onset of an atonic non-functioning colon and hypokalaemia, a condition marked by abnormally low levels of potassium in the blood, which otherwise usually occurs in dehydration.

Some of the more commonly prescribed stimulant laxatives include: *Bisacodyl tablets*; *Dulcolax* (manufacturers: Windsor); *Cascara tablets*; *Castor oil*; *Fig*; *Glycerol* (Glycerin); *Senna tablets*; *Manevac* (Galen); *Senokot* (Reckitt & Colman); *X-Prepp* (Napp).

FAECAL SOFTENERS – Probably the best known of these is *liquid paraffin* which can, however, often lead to anal irritation after prolonged use.

OSMOTIC LAXATIVES – These work by holding extra fluid in the bowel by osmosis or by altering the pattern of water distribution in the faeces. Some of these, particularly in the form of an enema, may be used to evacuate the bowel before certain radiological procedures or preceding endoscopy.

ANTISPASMODICS

Antispasmodics are drugs that relieve the spasm of smooth muscle, like those found in the gut, and are used quite frequently in the treatment of IBS as are other drugs that affect gut motility. There are several groups of these and the main ones are:

ANTIMUSCARINICS – One of the effects of these is to relax the oesophageal sphincter and a dose at night will usually delay gastric emptying, thereby prolonging the gastric retention of antacids which in turn helps reduce nocturnal acidity. Many of them are extremely strong drugs indeed and should be used with caution. Common side-effects associated with some of these include: difficulties in swallowing, dry mouth, thirst, increased intra-ocular pressure (which, of course, contra-indicates their use for patients suffering from glaucoma), difficulties in passing urine, constipation and dry skin.

Some commonly used antimuscarinics include: *Atropine sulphate* and *Belladonna alkaloids*; *Dicyclomine hydrochloride*; *Hyoscine butylbromide*; *Mepenzolate bromide*; *Pipenzolate bromide*; *Poldine methysulphate*; and *Propantheline bromide*.

Other antispasmodics include *Alverine citrate*, *Mebeverine hydrochloride*, and *peppermint oil*, all of which are credited with promoting the direct relaxation of intestinal smooth muscle and thereby relieving pain in IBS. None of these are associated with any serious side-effects, but – like all antispasmodics – should be avoided in cases of paralytic ileus, this being a condition where there is functional obstruction of the ileum, the lowest of the three portions of the small intestine. Paralytic ileum – which is also sometimes referred to as 'adynamic ileum' – may be caused by abdominal surgery, such as laparotomy, or may be the result of a deficiency of potassium in the blood or peritonitis.

Peppermint oil, which of course is also available as an over-the-counter remedy, is well-known for its ability to relieve abdominal colic and distension. Although it can be bought without a prescription, it really should only be used on the advice of your doctor as it should be used with caution. Heartburn and local irritation are two quite common side-effects. Preparations based on peppermint oil include: *Colpermin capsules* (manufacturers: Farmitalia) and *Mintec capsules* (Innovex).

SUMMING UP

Apart from those listed above, there are also many other types of medication used in the treatment of IBS. Many of these are, however, not so much of a treatment, but rather a temporary measure to provide transient relief from symptoms, such as the tranquillisers and anti-depressants that may be prescribed when anxiety or depression appears to be the root-cause of the problems. These, however, will be dealt with in the next chapter.

There is one more drug that may be prescribed and that is *Sodium cromoglycate* whose use is indicated in some types of food allergy when it is normally part of a programme that also involves dietary restrictions. Its side-effects include occasional nausea, rashes and possibly pain in the joints.

Chapter 8

The Mind And
Irritable Bowel Syndrome

TALKING ABOUT a 'vicious circle' may be using an otherwise over-worked cliché, but the phrase is never more apt than when it describes the interactions between the mental and physical well-being of many a sufferer from Irritable Bowel Syndrome.

The second phrase that automatically suggests itself is that of 'a chicken or egg' situation where there is little hope of discovering what might have come first – the physical symptoms of IBS or the worry and stress that accompany them? Or should that instead be 'cause' them?

While it may often be possible to determine whether stress brought on IBS in a given patient – or vice versa – it is just about impossible to generalise about this cause versus effect as far as the majority of sufferers in general are concerned. As with so many other aspects of IBS, the available evidence from various sources can be both contradictory and confusing. For example, if you were to ask a hundred doctors how much of a role stress plays in IBS, the answers would range from 'a great deal' to 'not as much as most people suppose'. And, no doubt, quite a few of those experts would add quite truthfully, 'we really don't know for sure'.

What all do seem to agree upon is that stress does affect not only how a particular individual may respond to the symptoms of IBS, but also how severe those symptoms can be as well as what course they may follow. Stress, of course, is something that everyone experiences at one time or another and in fact it is accepted as a truism that a certain amount of stress is needed by all of us. The difficulties arise when our level of stress exceeds that of our capability to cope with it. That is when this 'mental overload' may also express itself in many different kinds of physical manifestations, including those that are characteristic of IBS.

The above would seem to suggest that IBS is the 'chicken' in the chicken versus the egg equation. That is not necessarily the case because the other side of that coin, not to mix metaphors too much, is that IBS can also be the egg from which the chicken of stress hatches, as the painful and distressing symptoms of the syndrome also place a toll upon the emotional well-being of the sufferer. That leads us back to the vicious circle where one set of problems feeds upon another to exacerbate the situation as a whole.

In some ways the question of which comes first may not be all that important because on a practical level what matters is whether a given treatment brings improvement. It has been shown time and time again that:

☐ Treating a sufferer for stress may often relieve the IBS symptoms.
☐ Successfully treating a patient to relieve or reduce the typical IBS symptoms will also usually reduce stress levels.

In fact, these two separate approaches are often so intertwined that when progress is being made in solving one of the problems, the other almost invariably either disappears altogether or settles down to an acceptable level. You could say that it's almost a question of a vicious circle becoming a benign one.

What this means in practical terms is that the important thing is to break the vicious circle – whether this be accomplished by either relieving the IBS symptoms or reducing stress levels. There is a third, often simpler, approach which essentially consists not so much of reducing the levels of stress, but of using medication to make the stress more acceptable.

Which of these approaches is most likely to be successful will naturally enough depend upon the individual circumstances of a given case and one of the more difficult decisions that a doctor may have to make is to what extent stress needs to be dealt with as a separate entity that is deserving of treatment in its own right.

Sometimes, of course, it's pretty clear that the IBS symptoms are the result of a particularly stressful period. For example, should someone develop what appears to be IBS shortly after a bereavement, it's quite likely that the feelings of grief are manifesting themselves as physical problems. The digestive system seems to be particularly prone to reflect a state of mind as has been pointed out by Joe Macdonald Wallace, the Regional Director for Europe of the *International Stress and Tension Society*, who noted in his book 'Stress – A Practical Guide to Coping': "Acute stress has an immediate effect on appetite and digestive function. Chronic stress may lead to loss of appetite, irregular eating, gastric and duodenal ulcers, constipation or diarrhoea, or even ulcerative colitis. Any such changes may have a devastating effect on other bodily systems."

One of these systems often so affected is the excretory system which includes the end part of the alimentary canal. Added Mr Wallace: "Stress has an immediate effect on the functions of all these tissues and organs, and eventually on their structure, too. Any lack of efficiency in one of these organs is likely to have serious repercussions elsewhere."

It follows from the above that it is not uncommon for stress initially to provoke symptoms that are similar to those of IBS. Should the stress continue over a long enough period of time, this can actually cause structural changes in the digestive system. These changes may well lead to permanent symptoms which may remain long after the original stress factor – known, by the way, as a 'stressor' – has disappeared or dissipated.

ARE YOU SUFFERING FROM UNDUE STRESS?

The above is the logical question that will spring to the mind of many an IBS sufferer who will wonder whether all of his or her symptoms are indeed the result of stress. One of the big problems with stress is that it is a very difficult thing to quantify in the first instance and that becomes even more difficult when you consider the qualifying word 'undue' in the question posed above.

Let's look at what that elusive word 'stress' really means in this context. While there are many different definitions to be found in various medical and other dictionaries, the most helpful one is probably the one put forward by Dr Hans Selye, a world-renowned expert who has been credited with the discovery of the concept of biological stress. This is how he encapsulated his findings in his book 'Stress in Health and Disease': "Stress is the non-specific response of the body to any demand."

The key part of this definition, of course, is 'non-specific', in other words, a response that isn't necessary or vital to deal with the particular situation at hand. For example, developing an ache in your stomach isn't going to help you deal any better with a tough job interview, yet that is exactly what happens quite often.

So, in determining our individual stress levels, we have to be careful to separate those reactions which are needed to cope with or handle a demand and those which are superfluous and possibly harmful in the long-term. Some types of stress are in fact essential to our well-being as they are a vital and essential part of being alive. An extremely pleasant experience will also automatically generate a stress-type response, but – and this is the important part – will not add to 'undue' stress. It is the undue part that creates the problems.

Nevertheless, no matter how much we think we are in control of our emotions, we are all, to a greater or lesser degree, susceptible to undue stress, whether this is a result of over-reaction to events or because we have a low tolerance level in the first place. Once again, from a pragmatic point of view, it matters little which of these two main reasons is at work.

Going back to the original question of whether you are subject to undue levels of stress, there are many different types of psychological inventories which carefully allot points to different stressors and allow you to compare your score against a table which allegedly will indicate whether your level is high or low or somewhere in between. What, unfortunately, is not taken into account by these statistically-based inventories is the wide variation in the level of acceptable stress from person to person. An indication of how great this variation is can be found in a study by two American psychologists, Friess and Woolf, who came up with five main types of people, classifying these on the basis of their reaction to stimuli. The categories were:

☐ The 'hypoactive' personality – very little seems to affect these people who remain calm and detached under just about all circumstances and almost seem detached from whatever is happening around them.

☐ Then there were the three middle categories – comprising the 'calm', 'moderately active' and 'active'. These were people whose reactive patterns were broadly similar to those of the majority of the population.

☐ Finally, there was the 'hyperactive' type – people who were likely to respond strongly in an over-the-top way to almost all stimuli, as well as reacting emotionally to just about almost anything.

Further studies showed, not surprisingly, that the more active someone was in reaction to stimuli, the greater was the chance that their overall stress level would be in the 'undue' region. This means that when considering your own level of stress, you should first of all think about which of the above categories most nearly matches your own personality.

There is, of course, a much simpler – and often remarkably accurate – way of determining whether you're under undue stress and that is to ask yourself whether you are. If your answer is 'yes', the chances are that this is in fact the case. Equally, if you believe that you're not facing undue stress, once again your own assessment is likely to be the correct one.

For most of us, however, the answer is more likely to be somewhat equivocal, such as: "Well, I'm under stress, but not too much of it" or "Yes, I feel stressed, but I can cope with it" or "Some days I really feel that things are getting on top of me, but then there are other days when everything seems to be okay." If this sounds like you, the next question to consider is whether you've noticed any correlation between the times when you feel stressed and the occurrences of your IBS symptoms.

The link between the two may be quite obvious, such as when you know beforehand that your digestion is going to give you a tough time if you've had a hard day at the office, or you've noted that having an argument with someone is almost certain to be followed by a pain in the abdomen. In many instances, however, the connection between stress and IBS symptoms may not be all that obvious as there can be a considerable time-lag between the stressor and your worsening symptoms. This delay in effect following cause may be a matter of minutes, hours, days or even weeks as the stress may have to reach a cumulative plateau before it shows up as abdominal symptoms.

If you think that stress is causing your symptoms – or at least playing a major contributory role in provoking them – one of the ways you can verify this is by keeping a diary in which you note when stressors occur and also when you have particularly marked episodes of IBS. After doing this for a week or two, you may well be able to identify that there is a clearly defined link between the two and you may even be able to see what kind of stressors are particularly likely to bring on your physical symptoms. If you're really lucky, you may find that it is possible for you to avoid the worst stressors or eliminate them. For example, if you've found that you're always troubled badly by IBS the day after you've visited your in-laws, you may be able to reduce the number of times you see them. Or should you spot a pattern indicating that you invariably experience IBS symptoms three days after you've been to a party, you may choose to give this kind of social activity a miss for a while and see whether that helps.

Unfortunately, in most cases, although you may be able to identify the 'guilty' stressors, it may not be possible to avoid or eliminate them. Common stressors include such things as marital relationships, problems at work, worries about money – and it's not so easy to make that sort of problem simply go away. What can be done quite often, however, is to change your attitude to them and thereby make them less harmful to you in the long run. Especially useful in this connection are various relaxation and meditation techniques, some of which are explained in Chapter 10 of this book.

Another approach to dealing with stress is through medication. This, of course, will not actually reduce your stressors but will alter your reaction to them, thereby enabling you to gauge whether this also brings an improvement in your IBS symptoms over a period of time. Whether or not you should be prescribed drugs to relieve stress is, of course, a question for your doctor, but the way you choose to present your problems may well affect your doctor's decision.

The main clinical reasons for prescribing this sort of drug treatment are if your doctor is of the opinion that you are suffering from either anxiety or depression. Although these two conditions are so inter-linked that it can be extremely hard to diagnose which may be at work in an individual case, there are some specific guidelines – known as rating scales – which can give a strong indication. As a generality the symptoms of anxiety and depression can be compared as follows – this information being broadly based on the Montgomery and Asberg Depression Rating, the Hamilton Depression Rating Scale, and the Hamilton Anxiety Rating Scale, all of which are in common use:

□ **Symptoms seen in anxiety:** inner tension, difficulties in concentration and/or intellectual capacity, anxious mood, agitation, anxious signs and/or behaviour, gastrointestinal and/or genito-urinary disturbances, fears, psychic and somatic anxiety, as well as a variety of problems connected with the cardiovascular, respiratory and autonomic systems.

□ **Symptoms seen in depression:** sadness, inner tension, pessimistic thoughts and ideas, inability to feel emotions, reduced appetite and/or sleep, suicidal thoughts, guilt, loss of insight, difficulties in concentration, psychic and/or somatic anxiety, reduced sexual drive, as well as once again cardiovascular, autonomic and general somatic symptoms.

What is interesting about the two lists above is, first of all, that many of the symptoms appear in both, and, secondly, that gastrointestinal problems are specifically mentioned as part of the anxiety picture. However, as far as treatment goes, the situation is not quite so simple because, rather paradoxically, it has been found that quite often medication primarily intended to relieve depression does in fact do better in cases of anxiety than some drugs which were meant for that specific task. This naturally means that either or both types of drugs may possibly be used to treat anxiety. Bearing that possibility in mind, the following provides an outline of some of the main drug treatments which could be used to relieve anxiety caused by stress:

BENZODIAZEPINES. These drugs – of which *diazepam* and *lorazepam* are probably the best known and most widely prescribed examples – were first introduced in 1960 and are still nowadays considered to be the first line of defence against anxiety symptoms, despite the fact that in recent years the medical profession has become increasingly concerned by both the number of patients receiving the medication as well as the length of time they remained on it. Although the *Committee on Safety of Medicines* has recommended that benzodiazepines – while indicated for the short-term relief of severe or disabling anxiety – were to be considered as inappropriate and unsuitable for the treatment of short-term 'mild' anxiety, this recommendation has by no means been fully observed by many family doctors.

The main problem, of course, with these drugs is the high risk of dependence and the very serious difficulties that patients have had in coming off them. Despite that shortcoming, benzodiazepines continue to be frequently prescribed to alleviate comparatively mild anxiety and this may well be an approach that your family doctor may suggest if they believe that your IBS symptoms stem from stress levels which are high enough to create anxiety.

There are also some potential side-effects associated with the benzodiazepines and these, apart from the dependence risk already mentioned, include: drowsiness and/or light-headedness, headaches, vertigo, visual disturbances, rashes, and – of particular importance to IBS sufferers – gastrointestinal disturbances, although this last item is reported as occurring only occasionally. One intriguing aspect of the benzodiazepines is their ability to produce 'paradoxical' side-effects, that is effects which are actually the very contrary of what the drug might be expected to do. For example, patients on these medications have been known to show an increase in anxiety (as well as hostility or aggression, if these were present in the first place).

It is recommended that withdrawal from these drugs should usually be carried out gradually as abrupt cessation can produce a variety of symptoms, including many that are very similar to those which prompted them to be prescribed in the first instance. A typical protocol for this withdrawal process suggests that it takes place in fortnightly steps, the dosage being reduced to half the previous one at each step.

MAOIs. The initials stand for 'monoamine oxidase inhibitors'. Used in the treatment of both anxiety and depression, these drugs are known to be particularly efficient in treating so-called panic attacks. As a result they can be of particular relevance in IBS, where some patients have been able directly to connect their symptoms to such attacks. Great caution, however, needs to be exercised with these as they can interact dangerously with some foods as well as other drugs and for that reason their use is usually avoided when safer preparations are available.

ANTIDEPRESSANTS. As stated earlier, these can be more effective in the treatment of anxiety than those drugs meant specifically for that purpose. Another point in favour of the antidepressants is that there usually is a much smaller risk of dependency. On the debit side, however, antidepressants can be comparatively slow in producing their effects which may mean that some patients may not persevere with them long enough to gain any worthwhile benefit. Another problem with these drugs is that they have been known to create as side-effects some of the very symptoms that patients are most concerned about, such as irritability, insomnia and apprehension.

It's clear from the above that, despite the often heard claims from the pharmaceutical industry, there really are no 'wonder' drugs that will solve all problems. Many medications will indeed do a great job of providing a relatively stress-free period and this can be extremely useful if the patient needs a 'breathing space' in which to sort out his or her problems. But there always is a downside attached to the potential benefits, including the chances of unpleasant side-effects and/or dependence. While it is up to your doctor to decide whether they are willing to prescribe these preparations, it is also up to you to decide whether you in fact wish to take them.

The above is not to be construed as suggesting that the psychoactive drugs should be avoided as they have indeed proven time and time again their worth in helping to control or reduce the symptoms of IBS when these were the result of stress. But their benefit only lasts as long as you take them and, sooner or later, you will wish to stop using them. If by then you've been able to sort out whatever was putting you under undue stress and making your symptoms appear, all well and good. If your situation, however, is still very much like it was before you began taking the medication, then all you might have gained is some time at the possible cost of having to face withdrawal or dependency problems.

Fortunately, there are other ways of dealing with stress than just by medication and this is the subject to which the next two chapters are devoted.

Chapter 9

Psychotherapy And Hypnotherapy Treatments In IBS

HAVING SEEN in previous chapters how closely emotional states and Irritable Bowel Syndrome symptoms are linked in some patients, it's not surprising that the medical profession has sought to cure IBS by using methods that address the psychological factors instead of the physical ones.

Essentially, these methods fall into one of three main groups: psychotherapy, hypnotherapy, and group management clinics where patients are taught techniques to control their own stress levels. Although these approaches are comparatively new and are at this time only available in certain specialist centres, they are indicative of how well treatments which look at curing the body by affecting the mind can do in cases of IBS. In most instances, of course, these kind of treatments are only offered to patients whose IBS symptoms are refractory, that is they don't respond well – or not at all – to other and more conventional therapies.

Explaining the rationale behind the idea of adopting psychotherapeutic methods for dealing with refractory IBS patients, Dr Else Guthrie, of the Manchester Royal Infirmary, stated at a recent conference of gastroenterologists, psychiatrists and psychologists: "This has developed from three main areas. First, there is a substantial psychoanalytic literature on the relationship between somatic symptomatology and emotional conflict. Secondly, many studies have noted a relationship between the irritable bowel syndrome and psychological factors. Finally, a small number of controlled treatment studies employing a variety of psychological methods have produced encouraging results."

As evidence of how effective psychotherapeutic treatment can be, Dr Guthrie provided details of a recent, randomised, controlled trial conducted at her hospital. Although originally 115 patients were considered for the study, this number was eventually whittled down to 102 as several were dropped for a variety of reasons, including two who couldn't speak English, and five who had severe depression with suicidal ideation.

The patients recruited into the study were all sufferers from 'severe' IBS symptoms which they had had continuously for longer than a year and they had also been attending a specialist gastrointestinal clinic for at least six months previously without showing any improvement. For the actual trial, the patients were divided into two groups which were broadly similar in age, marital status, types of jobs, and social class. By the end of the study, because of some more patients dropping out and others being diagnosed as having specific physical problems, the total number involved had dropped to 96, 50 in a treatment group and 46 in a control group.

Some indication of how marked the IBS symptoms were in the members of these groups can be gleaned from the following: the average duration of continuous symptoms was two years (ranging from one to twenty years); more than 40 per cent of them had been seen by at least three different consultant gastroenterologists; two out of five had been admitted to hospital for investigation on at least two separate occasions; and the 56 patients who were in employment had been forced to take off an average of six weeks' sick leave within the last year because of IBS.

The actual study was carried out over a period of 12 weeks during which time each member of the treatment group received a total of seven sessions of psychotherapy: one long introductory session at first which was then followed by six more shorter ones spread throughout the length of the study. The specific approach used in these sessions was based on the assumption that the patient's problems originally arose from disturbances in significant personal relationships. Aspects of these disturbances were then re-enacted during treatment in the relationship between the patient and the therapist and, if this developed in a healthy way, this should have allowed the patient to make connections between their emotional conflicts and symptoms.

Explaining this further, Dr Guthrie added: "The psychotherapist does not attempt to force a psychological explanation of physical symptoms on to the patient, but merely tries to help the patient to understand and acknowledge any emotional factors that seem relevant to the physical symptoms that he/she is experiencing."

In contrast to the group being treated, the control group instead received five sessions of what was described as 'supportive listening' in which the doctor, although warm and sympathetic to the problems, did not attempt either to create an 'intense' relationship with the patient nor to analyse any relationship that might have been tentatively in the process of being formed. In other words, these sessions merely gave the patient a sympathetic hearing of their difficulties, much as might have been provided by any caring non-psychotherapeutically qualified person.

At the end of the trial, all patients were extensively tested to find out whether there had been any improvement or changes and this is what the researchers found:

☐ As far as gastrointestinal symptoms were concerned, the members of the treatment group had significantly improved in a variety of ways. They reported fewer incidences of abdominal pain than before; and the pain they reported was broadly speaking less severe than it had been. Overall, these patients also found that the limiting effect that their symptoms had previously imposed on their daily lives had been substantially reduced. Although the results outlined above could be interpreted by some as not being objective enough as they depended to a large extent upon the patients' own assessments, these improvements were also confirmed by gastroenterologists.

☐ A similar overall improvement was also noted for the treatment group when their psychological symptoms were assessed at the end of the trial, using a variety of measures, such as the Beck Depression Inventory, the Symptom Rating Test and the Psychiatric Assessment Schedule. Most important, as far as the researchers were concerned, was the fact that the improvement in gastrointestinal functions 'correlated significantly' with changes in psychological symptoms score. In other words, as the treatment only addressed psychological factors and yet yielded more or less matching physical improvements, it was clear from this that the value of this psychotherapeutic approach was proven and that this was definitely superior to 'supportive listening'.

When the results were analysed further, some additional facts emerged:

☐ The psychotherapy had worked better with women than with men.

☐ The majority of female patients had maintained their improvement when they were followed up a year later. There was a similar trend for the men, but the data wasn't solid enough to be considered conclusive.

☐ Although all the patients in the study had chronic IBS, those who had complained of other symptoms which were not typical of IBS, such as constant pain, did not as a whole respond as well as those with classical IBS symptoms.

☐ The presence of psychiatric illness in a patient usually meant that there would be a good response to the treatment.

☐ There was also a marked difference in response between those patients who had complained of constant pain in that the treatment did little to ease their symptoms. On the other hand, those patients who from the outset had thought that their symptoms were exacerbated by stress did well.

Taking all the findings into account, this study – which is broadly representative of other similar ones – does demonstrate very clearly how changing a patient's outlook can bring direct physical benefits. While this sort of psychotherapeutic treatment which, of course, places great demands upon the health service, is not likely to become available in the near future to all who might need it, it does nevertheless provide proof that other, less expensive to provide, psychological approaches aimed at reducing stress may often be a viable alternative therapy for IBS.

A possible long-term answer might lie in a comparatively new technique called *group stress management* which – because it doesn't involve the doctor on a one-to-one basis – is a good deal cheaper to provide. An interesting clinical trial to compare the effectiveness of such a programme against that of drug-based treatment was recently concluded at the Gloucester Royal Hospital. The study was random in that the patients were chosen consecutively from those attending out-patient gastroenterologist clinics and the final sample consisted of six men and thirty-one women, aged from 19 to 67 years (average age, 40), who had all experienced comparatively severe IBS symptoms for at least six months to as long as twenty years. After a series of interviews and assessments, the patients were split into two groups by random allocation.

The first group was treated by a 'psychological management programme', this consisting essentially of six sessions – each attended by five to eight patients – of ninety minutes' duration. Each session consisted of a talk of about 15 minutes, followed by discussion, a break for coffee, and then another 15-minute talk, a relaxation session, and a final summary. Typical subjects covered in the talks were: What is IBS?; The role of stress in IBS; Progressive muscle relaxation; Using relaxation constructively; Diet and fitness; Long-term management of IBS; and, Problem solving.

During the same six-week-long period, the second group was treated by conventional pharmacological means, including the following medications as required: *Motival* (a compound antidepressant preparation), antispasmodics, antidiarrhoeals and/or bulking agents.

After the treatment schedule was completed, the members of both groups were examined at the out-patients' clinic where they were assessed once more. A further follow-up assessment was carried out six months later after which the findings were analysed. This is what the researchers discovered:

☐ In general, both the physical and psychological symptoms of patients in both groups had been reduced by treatment, and these reductions reached statistical significance in many instances.

☐ While the differences between the two groups weren't all that marked immediately after treatment, these became apparent six months thereafter when the follow-up assessment showed that psychology had quite dramatically outperformed pharmacology. In particular, it was noted that many of the drug-treated patients were rapidly slipping back towards their original pre-treatment levels of IBS symptoms, despite the fact that nearly all of them were still taking the prescribed medications.

Summing up the findings, Dr Nichola Rumsey, of Bristol Polytechnic, who was the research psychologist for the trial, stated: "The results indicate that for this sample (of patients), group psychological management was a successful, if not preferable, alternative to a conventional pharmacological treatment."

Explaining why she thought that the treatment had worked so well, Dr Rumsey provided the following reasons:

1) The programme was received favourably by the patients who took part in it.

2) Many patients obviously enjoyed being part of a group.

3) Many of the patients found the relaxation techniques which were taught particularly helpful.

4) Some patients liked the increase in feelings of control over their condition associated with it.

5) The information on how to deal with stress was welcomed by many.

6) Many found that the programme had increased their self-confidence.

Additionally, 78 per cent of the patients said that the medical teaching they had received about IBS had been 'very' to 'extremely' useful, and 75 per cent reported the same level of satisfaction with what they had learned about the connections between stress, anxiety, tension and IBS. The highest score, however, was obtained in answer to the question "Was it worth coming on the course?" to which 86 per cent said "yes".

Once again, the above proves – as with one-to-one psychotherapy – that a treatment approach which is purely addressed to the mind can work wonders in IBS even in those cases which have a long history of ongoing severe symptoms. This ability of psychological techniques to provide relief where other methods had failed in the past was also underlined by another important study where hypnosis was used to achieve results that were remarkable by any standard.

The patients involved in this study at the University Hospital in South Manchester were once again those who had had IBS symptoms for a long time and these had proven to be refractory to normal treatments. Initially, there was a comparatively small trial involving 30 patients who were chosen at random either to receive psychotherapy or hypnotherapy, the latter consisting of a total of seven sessions of thirty minutes each over three months. Summing up the findings of this first study, Dr Alison Prior and Dr P J Whorwell, who had conducted it, stated: "At the end of the three months the hypnotherapy group showed a dramatic response with almost complete resolution of symptoms."

These results were, of course, so encouraging that it was decided to explore hypnotherapy further and since then about 200 patients have been treated for IBS in that way by four different hypnotherapists. The gratifying results have continued to pour in with the latest figures showing an overall favourable response rate of 80 per cent, much higher than the success rate usually obtained with more traditional treatments.

Here's how the hypnotherapy is provided. To begin with, the patient is given a brief explanation of how the gut works and also given some practical insight into the concept of abnormal gut sensitivity. Thereafter, one of several standard methods of inducing hypnosis is used, this usually being one that involves the so-called 'eye fixation technique' in which the subject is asked to fix their attention on a finger or a hand.

When the patient reaches a hypnotic state, the therapist then suggests the progressive relaxation of various muscle groups to deepen the hypnosis. Often much of the first session is spent on induction and relaxation, but a suggestion is implanted at this time to make the induction process much faster in later sessions.

The relaxation component of the hypnotherapeutic treatment is then followed by what the doctors call the 'gut directed' therapy which has two main aspects. Firstly, the patient is asked to identify the part of the abdomen which is most painful, place their hand on it and then to 'feel' warmth coming from that hand into the abdomen and to associate this with relief from pain and muscular spasm. Thereafter, the patient is asked to visualise this as a way of pinpointing the origin of the symptoms and also how to get rid of them. For example, in a specific case where the main IBS symptom is that of diarrhoea, the subject might be led into seeing his bowel as a fast-flowing stream which gradually loses its speed until all the turbulence disappears. The therapist will then try to use this tranquil image as something against which the patient can 'reset' their visualisation of their bowel.

At the conclusion of each session, the patient is given some ego-bolstering suggestions – such as 'You're going to do well' or 'You'll feel fine' – all of these carrying a positive message that things are already getting better.

The treatment is reinforced at about the halfway point when the patient is given an audio tape which they can listen to and use for further relaxation and visualisation on a daily basis at home. The doctors pointed out: "Hypnosis will not work for the patients who think that they can come along once a week and passively wait for some magical experience to happen." They also emphasised that as they were not trained psychiatrists, they never attempted hypno-analysis during the sessions and didn't even seek to discuss stress factors with the patients while they were under hypnosis.

Despite these limitations, the study has produced some impressive results, particularly with patients suffering from classical IBS symptoms, of which a staggering 95 per cent responded favourably, that is with their symptoms either becoming markedly milder or disappearing altogether.

Patients whose symptoms were not typically characteristic of IBS – such as those who had abdominal pain without either distension or changes in bowel habits – did, however, fare much worse as a group with only 45 per cent of them responding favourably. It was also found that in general those subjects who showed high levels of anxiety or depression also did less well as did those older than 55 years even when their symptoms were the classical ones.

From these statistics, it's clear that the treatment works. But how does it do so? The doctors admitted they themselves didn't quite know, saying: "It is almost impossible to elucidate how hypnotherapy works ... There is such a complex inter-relationship between the brain and the gut that it is impossible to determine at which level the hypnosis may be acting."

This inability to state exactly how a given treatment achieves its results is, of course, something that is encountered quite frequently in IBS, the main point remaining that success ensues a particular course of action. Unfortunately, as with so many other promising treatments, hypnotherapy is time-consuming and expensive to provide and therefore is generally limited to those patients who have severe problems which have proven refractory to other therapies. One way of reducing the cost is by providing hypnotherapy on a group basis with several patients receiving treatment simultaneously, rather like the group stress management study mentioned above. Although this has been successful in several trials, it doesn't quite produce the same degree of improvement as does the much more intensive one-to-one therapy.

Cost-effectiveness remains a big factor in IBS treatment and with a National Health Service that is faced with tremendous financial pressures from all sides, this is likely to remain so in the foreseeable future. This means that the more expensive treatments are unlikely to be made available for many sufferers of IBS who might well have benefited from them. However, while all of the above has been concerned with psychological approaches provided by highly-skilled and trained professionals to treat IBS symptoms, some of the very same principles that underly these expensive therapies can sometimes be used by the patients themselves through various relaxation and meditation techniques. It is these we'll look at in the next chapter.

Chapter 10

How Relaxation Techniques Can Help

I N PREVIOUS chapters we have seen firstly, that stress and tension can often provoke the symptoms of Irritable Bowel Syndrome and, secondly, that various treatments which are based on dealing solely with psychological factors can often greatly reduce the severity of these symptoms and even make them disappear altogether.

From this it follows that relaxation techniques – a phrase which in its broadest sense can also include meditation – can often help reduce your IBS problems by acting in two very different yet interlinked ways:

1) You can use relaxation to prevent your stress and tension levels reaching such a point that they cause your IBS symptoms to appear. This is relaxation as a preventative measure.

2) You can also use relaxation to help reduce the intensity of symptoms which have already appeared. This is relaxation as a means of providing relief from pain or discomfort.

Although these two approaches to dealing with your symptoms are quite different, the specific techniques that are used in either case are very similar, with the main difference being in when and how you use them.

Most sufferers from IBS will, of course, gain the greatest benefit by using relaxation as needed both for prevention and relief. Ideally, the preventative aspect of stress control will be powerful enough to avoid symptoms from emerging. Should that fail to do the job fully, however, then such symptoms as do occur – and these hopefully will already do so in a less severe form than they might have otherwise – may then be eased by further relaxation exercises.

The basic principle behind all generally used relaxation programmes is extremely simple and essentially amounts to saying: "If the body can be brought to a state of physical relaxation, then the mind, too, will become relaxed, dissipating stress and tension." The paramount importance of this physical relaxation is well recognised by the medical profession as, for example, shown by the study described in the previous chapter where group stress management classes also placed great emphasis on physical relaxation.

The idea that mental and physical relaxation are two sides of one coin is not all that new and it is now accepted as an absolute fact that thinking is not merely a matter for the mind, but is also directly connected with both voluntary and involuntary contractions of the muscles in various parts of your body. This two-way traffic between your thought processes and your actions is illustrated in all sorts of situations: if your mind is tense as you concentrate on a tough exam, the chances are your back, neck and leg muscles will be so as well; if you become excited while watching a sporting event, this excitement will also be reflected in physical excitement, such as possibly exhibited by waving your arms or jumping up and down as your team scores a goal; and feelings of deep anger will usually also make you talk louder, tighten up your face and clench your whole body.

On the other hand, the reverse is equally true. If you're sitting comfortably and quietly having pleasant thoughts, your body will also soon reflect that inner tranquillity by assuming a relaxed pose in which the muscles have the minimum amount of tenseness to keep you safely in your position.

It perhaps needs to be stressed that the idea of using the body to relax the mind – or vice versa – is not the product of some kind of mysticism, or any other 'ism' for that matter. It is an idea that has been proven beyond doubt by countless experimental studies, many of which have specifically demonstrated the very strong links between emotional states and the digestive system as a whole and the symptoms of IBS in particular. The big trick, of course, is how to use this information so that by relaxing your body you quieten your mind and this in turn provides a beneficial soothing effect upon your digestive system.

A BASIC TECHNIQUE

We'll begin by looking at a very basic technique which can be used by just about anyone on a daily basis – or even more frequently – to lay the groundwork for a more specific programme later when you've mastered this one.

First of all, seek out a time of the day when you can reasonably expect that you won't be interrupted by others, the doorbell or the telephone, perhaps taking the latter off the hook for the duration of your relaxation period. It will also probably help if you can wear clothing that is nice and loose and doesn't constrict you. If it's not possible to change to such clothing, then at least loosen anything – like a belt, bra or tie – which might interfere with your body relaxing fully.

You begin this relaxation exercise by lying down comfortably. This can be either on the floor or on a bed. If it's the bed, don't choose one that has a very soft mattress into which your body sinks too much. If it makes you feel more comfortable, place a light support under your head, such as a rolled up towel or small cushion.

Lie down flat on your back with your legs fully extended and slightly spread apart and your arms more or less by your sides but also spreading out slightly. According to personal preference, you may choose to have the palms of your hands either pointing up or down.

Slowly, without any hurry, gradually seek to clear your mind of any extraneous thoughts that may be there and make it as blank as possible. Then alternatively contract – that is tense up – and deliberately relax various groups of muscles throughout your body.

It is very important that you contract a given muscle before you relax it and don't just try to relax from what might be a semi-tense state. By tensing up first, you'll experience and learn to recognise the contrast between a tense and a relaxed muscle. One way of ensuring that you contract the muscle fully is to tense it for at least ten seconds or so as the tenseness then builds up to its full extent. After a count of ten seconds, relax the muscle by consciously letting go, leaving the muscle to go limp and resting wherever it is supported only by gravity.

This 'tense up, then relax' procedure is carried out sequentially for each major set of muscles in your body until you've dealt with all of them. Although you could probably relax the muscles in any order you might like and still benefit, there is a sequence which works best for most people and which gradually works its way from the extremities to the head. This is the recommended order in which you should contract and relax the various muscles:

- ☐ Begin with the toes, as these represent the point furthest away from your head, and try to do each toe individually. Then move on to the feet, one at a time, and move upwards to deal with the calves, knees, thighs and buttocks. Alternate between left and right sides until all parts of both of your legs are fully relaxed.

- ☐ Then move on to the trunk, beginning by contracting and relaxing the lower abdomen, then the upper abdomen, the lower back, the upper back, the chest and finally the shoulders. For IBS sufferers, it can be particularly useful really to concentrate on getting the maximum amount of relaxation in all the muscles in the abdomen. One of the ways of ensuring that you achieve this is by doing a series of contraction and relaxation cycles when you're working on this area. Please note that while the idea is initially to tense up as much as you can, you should not of course do this to the point where it actually hurts, merely to the extent where you can feel the muscles as tense as they can be before any actual pain or severe discomfort is felt.

- ☐ The next stage is to concentrate on the arms. Begin with the fingers, one at a time, then the hands, the wrists, the forearm, the elbow, the upper arm, and just for luck do the shoulders once more as these are often reluctant to loosen up completely the first time around.

☐ Next on the list are the neck and the head. Begin with the neck, moving this slightly sideways if that helps, then the throat, the lower jaw, the face – that is chin, lips, cheeks, nose, forehead and the eyes. Do the eyes by tightening and relaxing your eyelids and also gently moving your eyes from side to side as well as up and down.

☐ When you've relaxed all your muscles, just lie still for some ten minutes or so, letting the feeling of relaxation spread all over your body while you clear your mind of all worries and problems. Feel yourself sinking down into the floor or the bed as your whole body continues to unwind. Many people say that thinking of peaceful images – such as clouds slowly drifting across the sky or of green fields – will help them relax even more at this time. Be aware of the rhythm of your breathing and notice how it slows down as you relax more deeply.

☐ Remain lying still for at least ten minutes to gain the full benefit, all the time keeping your mind as tranquil as your body.

☐ When your allotted time is up, don't suddenly get up, but do this gently and slowly, using a series of movements that gradually return the needed tension to your muscles until you're moving normally once again.

Ideally, you should seek to perform the above relaxation pro-gramme every day. Don't expect too much from it the first couple of times that you do it as it can take a while for the benefits to build up and also for you to get used to the sequence of relaxing the various muscle groups in turn. However, after you've done this a couple of times or more, you'll soon find that the sequence goes, as it were, on 'automatic pilot' and you won't even have to think about it any more.

If, however, you find that after a while you still do have to concentrate on what bit comes next and this interferes with your mental relaxation, you can solve this problem by making a simple tape recording on which you just speak the key words 'toes', 'ankles', etc, at suitably timed intervals. Playing back the tape will then provide your cues.

The above exercise is, of course, a very simple one whose main aim is to induce relief from stress and tension generally by creating a relaxed mind and body. It could well be that this is in fact enough already to produce a great improvement in your IBS symptoms, but in many instances you may need to be more specific in your approach.

How you make your relaxation exercises 'symptom specific' is a matter for trial and error as no two people have exactly the same circumstances or have identical reactions or symptoms. Here are some ways that have been successfully used by others in similar situations:

☐ When you've reached the final relaxation state at the end of the exercise, spend some time mentally exploring your gut, using whatever imagery you find apt to match your own symptoms. For example, if constipation is one of your problems, picture in your mind a dam that's blocking a river's natural flow; then see the dam slowly disintegrate to release the stream.

☐ If acute discomfort in one or more specific parts of your abdomen is one of your main symptoms, visualise the areas where the pain is most common as being overheated or on fire. Think of fresh water spraying on these areas, cooling them down or damping the fire.

☐ If diarrhoea is one of your IBS symptoms, you may find it helpful to invoke images like cement being added to water to make a more solid mix; or mud drying out under the sun after a rainfall.

☐ In most people's minds, warmth – but not heat – is synonymous with comfort and healing and you can use this link as you visualise a therapeutic feeling of warmth gently permeating your whole digestive system and easing discomfort wherever it reaches.

The use of the power of the mind to create images that engender bodily reactions is a well-documented phenomenon and this is exactly what makes it possible for hypnotherapy to achieve the high rates of success in treating IBS described earlier. You can, by using your own imagination, also draw upon this power to achieve worthwhile results.

Going hand in hand with relaxation is the principle of meditation which is not, as some might suppose, a mystic idea but merely a way of dealing with your thoughts and allowing you to gain control over those that otherwise would make you feel tense, anxious or agitated. Additionally, meditation is a technique that permits you to explore your own mind in a calm and free-flowing way that nevertheless can be aimed at producing specific results.

As with physical relaxation, meditation is most likely to bring benefits if carried out regularly, preferably daily. Once again, don't expect too much from your first few sessions, but carry on until the meditative approach becomes automatic and natural to you.

While there is no specific way in which you should sit or lie to meditate, it's obviously important that you should be at ease and comfortable, whether sitting in an easy chair or lying down. It's usually best to start with some physical relaxation first and carrying out an abbreviated form of the programme outlined earlier will generally be helpful.

Once you've reached a state of physical relaxation, start the meditative process by one of the following methods:

□ Close your eyes and think about your breathing rhythm; don't concentrate on it as such, but merely become aware of the natural inhalation and exhalation process, saying mentally to yourself 'one' each time you breathe out and 'two' as you breathe in. As the minutes go by, you'll find your breathing rate slows down and your whole body relaxes even further. After a few more minutes, stop saying 'one' and 'two' to yourself and just sit there quietly for a little while longer, keeping your eyes closed and your mind as blank as possible, basking in the total relaxation of your mind and body.

☐ After having once again first achieved physical relaxation, close your eyes and choose to let your mind travel to a place (either real or imaginary) where you'd like to be, such as a warm beach, a pleasant village, a sunlit meadow, whatever strikes your fancy. Use your mind's eye to explore all the facets of this wonderful and peaceful place, its sights, sounds and smells, as you delight in your presence there. After a while, slowly return your mind to where you are, remembering the sense of peace and inner calm you felt as you visited that other place.

☐ Once again, while physically relaxed, look in-depth at an object that really pleases you – this could be a vase of flowers, a statuette, a painting, even a brightly-coloured and especially beautiful leaf. Bring all your senses to bear on this object, your eyes seeking out every intricate detail of its contours, your mind responding to each pattern it recognises, and your hands feeling its shape and texture. After concentrating like this for a while, close your eyes and recreate the object in your mind and think about all its beautiful aspects.

☐ If you have a clock with a moderately loud ticking noise, you can use this as an aid to launch you into a meditative state. Close your eyes when you're physically relaxed and let your mind concentrate on the regularity of the alternating 'ticks' and 'tocks', letting these lull you into feelings of serenity and calm. You might also begin by mentally saying to yourself 'tick' and 'tock' to match the clock's perpetual rhythm and then, as you relax further, simply listening to it until you're no longer even aware of it.

As you can see from the above, there are many different ways to achieve a meditative state and you'll perhaps have to experiment somewhat to find out for yourself which one works best for you. As is so often the case with other things, the key to success is perseverance: if at first you don't succeed, do try again.

The purpose of reaching a meditative state is three-fold:

☐ Firstly, this meditative state helps you achieve a sense of inner peace and tranquillity which has a damping-down effect on the stressors you encounter as part of your daily life.

☐ Secondly, it can be used as a way to counteract the stresses of a particularly tense day or event.

☐ Thirdly, and this can be the most important part of all as far as IBS sufferers are concerned, once you get used to meditating and find it easy to get yourself in a meditative state, you can use this as a way of reinforcing the various images that you had previously used during relaxation to control IBS symptoms. How you do this is by conjuring up these thoughts at the end of a meditation session when your state of mind will be such that it will be more receptive to them and they therefore are more likely to bring the actual physical benefits you're seeking.

There is another technique that is often used as part of either relaxation or meditation. That is breath control which, apart from helping you relax, can also help revitalise your body as a whole, because the extra intake of oxygen 'recharges' your whole organism.

The single most useful breath control exercise is what is known as the *Complete Breath*. This is a technique that has been derived from ancient Hatha Yoga, which is the name of that part of the Yoga discipline concerned with controlling physical matters.

An excellent time to practise the Complete Breath is at the end of your relaxation exercises while you're still lying down. Here's what you do:

1) Gently bring your legs and feet together.

2) Take in a deep breath and at the same time raise your arms upwards making the hands meet above your head and then move them further back so that your arms end up lying straight out behind your head with their palms facing up.

3) Now exhale slowly and bring your arms back to where they originally were, by your sides.

4) Repeat the same procedure up to about ten times in all, letting each cycle flow smoothly into the next one. Bear

in mind that the movements should not be rushed and should be as smooth as possible.

If circumstances don't allow you to lie down, you can also use the Complete Breath as a pick-me-up while standing and without necessarily having gone through a relaxation session first. This is what you do:

1) Stand relaxed, keeping your back straight with your head erect and looking straight in front of you, your feet and legs together with the feet pointing slightly apart for better balance. Your arms should be hanging loosely by your sides with your hands, their palms turned into your body, brushing your upper thighs.

2) Take in a deep breath while you gradually bring your arms up sideways with the palms turning so they are uppermost. Continue raising your arms in a smooth movement until the hands meet above your head with your arms pointing straight up.

3) Let your breath come out slowly as you bring your arms back to where they were, by your sides.

4) Repeat the above up to ten times.

SUMMING UP

The various exercises and techniques described above, of course, cover only a very small number of the various ways in which both relaxation and meditation can be used to bring about improvements in physical complaints such as IBS. However, it may well be that the few simple programmes outlined above – and adapted by yourself to suit your specific needs – may be enough to bring relief.

Finally, it's worth stating that even if at the end of the day relaxation and meditation don't help you with your IBS symptoms, it could well be that they may nevertheless provide other health benefits. For that reason alone it's certainly worth giving them a try, as there is little to lose and possibly a great deal to gain.

The medical profession as a whole endorses the idea of relaxation training and therefore it's not really what might be called an alternative therapy as such. There are, however, many alternative therapies which have proven successful in dealing with IBS and so it is these we will look at in the next chapter.

Chapter 11

Alternative Medicine Treatments For Irritable Bowel Syndrome

MANY IRRITABLE Bowel Syndrome sufferers end up eventually seeking help from practitioners of alternative forms of medicine. The reasons for this are both many and complex, but some of the main ones, according to a recent survey, include:

☐ Some patients feel that their family doctors don't treat them with the seriousness that they feel their symptoms deserve. Their doctors are often somewhat dismissive of IBS once it's been proven to be 'nothing more serious' and reluctant to spend too much time dealing with it if the symptoms are only moderately severe.

☐ IBS is often a chronic problem whose symptoms wax and wane in both severity and frequency for no particularly obvious or easily explained reasons. Traditional Western medicine is by no means always successful in dealing with these ongoing and changing problems and this makes sufferers wonder whether there might be something to be gained from other therapies.

☐ As IBS, by definition, seems to lack an obvious physical cause in most instances and its occurrence is frequently strongly linked to emotional states, patients may conclude that alternative treatments which often focus their attention on the 'whole' person may be more efficient in providing a solution.

☐ Not unreasonably, patients may also seek out alternative practitioners because they are desperate for improvement and this doesn't seem to be forthcoming from conventional medicine, despite having tried all it had to offer them.

While these are all good reasons for considering finding out what alternative medicine might have to offer, there is also a need to be cautious. While most practitioners are highly trained and reputable, there is unfortunately a fringe element whose ethical and professional standards can be lacking. Although it is sensible to be careful in choosing an alternative medicine practitioner, this shouldn't stop you from seeing one if that is what you want to do. However, make your choice from those who are accredited to a professional body of some standing. Personal recommendation from someone whose judgement you trust can also be a good guide. And although medical doctors aren't supposed to recommend alternative practitioners, you just might have a doctor who is prepared at least to offer a comment which you then might have to interpret fully for yourself.

It also goes without saying – although said it will be – that before seeking help elsewhere you should certainly see your own doctor initially to ensure that a proper diagnosis is made first, if only to exclude other possible causes for your symptoms. You should also go back to your doctor if you were to develop any new symptoms or if your existing ones were to become more severe while you are being treated by someone else.

Which of the many alternative forms of therapy might be worth a try is really a matter of individual choice, as all of them have their ardent supporters. Here to help you make your choice are details of the main ones.

ACUPUNCTURE

This is based on the ages old Oriental medical system that was first developed in China. The therapy works by using needles – or sometimes other objects – to stimulate specific points on the body and this in turn creates beneficial changes elsewhere in the body. One of the aims of this system is to 'rebalance forces' and thereby improve the health of the subject as whole as well as provide treatment for specific ailments that are present.

Acupuncturists subscribe to the ancient Chinese philosophy that states that there is a life force – known as 'chi' – which is made up of negative and positive flows of energy, respectively called 'yin' and 'yan', which course throughout the body along channels which are known as 'meridians'. Disease and pain are seen as the results of an interruption or an imbalance in these flows of energy. Stimulation by acupuncture is meant to restore the normal and healthy flow along the meridians.

One of the better known and more commonly used forms of alternative medicine in the West, acupuncture has a long and proven record in being particularly effective in relieving pain. It is also an alternative therapy that has gained a fair degree of acceptance from conventional medicine and is quite frequently used by doctors.

While there is much controversy about how acupuncture works – one popular theory suggests that the needles cause the body to release additional 'endorphins', which are natural pain killers – there is little doubt that it certainly has been an effective treatment for some IBS sufferers.

For the squeamish who may be put off by the very idea of having needles inserted into their body, it's worth pointing out that the procedure is not in the slightest bit painful and at worst might be slightly uncomfortable.

It's naturally best to consult a qualified acupuncturist and you can get more information from: *The British Medical Acupuncture Society*, Newton House, Newton Lane, Lower Whitley, Warrington, Cheshire WA4 4JA; *The Council for Acupuncture*, 179 Gloucester Place, London NW1 6DX; *The Association of Chinese Acupuncture* (College of Oriental Medicine), Prospect House, 2 Grove Lane, Retford, Nottingham DN22 6NA; *The British Acupuncture Association*, 34 Alderney Street, London SW1V 4EU; *The Register of Chinese Medicine*, 19 Trinity Road, London N2 8JJ; or *The Traditional Acupuncture Society*, 11 Grange Park, Stratford-upon-Avon, Warwickshire CV37 6HX.

ACUPRESSURE

This works on broadly the same principle as acupuncture with the essential difference between the two being that the various points in the body are massaged by the practitioner's finger or thumb instead of using needles. One of the advantages of this method is that a patient may well be taught to be able to perform this massage for themself and therefore continue the treatment as needs be on their own. Most practitioners of acupuncture also offer acupressure therapy as some patients cannot face the idea of having needles stuck into them. For more information contact the acupuncturist groups listed above.

HOMOEOPATHY

Almost without a doubt the most generally accepted form of alternative medicine, homoeopathy is a treatment system developed in the late 1700s by Samuel Hahnemann. It is based on two essential principles: firstly, that 'like cures like'; and, secondly, that 'less is more'. Homoeopaths also believe that symptoms are signs which are produced by the body's efforts to resist or throw off infection or disease.

Homoeopathic practitioners claim that the body can cope with most illnesses and that the doctor's main job is to help strengthen its innate ability to heal itself. To aid and stimulate the body's natural defences in that task, treatment is usually administered in extremely small doses of various preparations, these being taken either as tablets or as liquids, which are prepared from natural substances and originating from various herbal, animal, mineral and metallic sources. Another of the guiding principles of homoeopathy is that of 'Minimal Dose' – that is that the smallest possible amount of the indicated active ingredient should be prescribed – and in practice this means that the remedies are supplied in a form that is so diluted that often none of the original healing ingredient can still be detected in the final mixture. For sceptics, this naturally enough raises the question of how can a remedy possibly have any therapeutic effect if there is nothing – or very little – left of the main substance? Homoeopathic practitioners admit freely that they, too, don't know why the remedies should work, but point with pride to the accumulated evidence that seems to prove beyond doubt that it does. The efficacy of homoeopathy has been endorsed time and time again after being subjected to the most stringent tests.

Like acupuncture, homoeopathy is an alternative therapy that is also used quite frequently by some medically qualified doctors and, under certain circumstances, it is even available free through the National Health Service.

You don't need a prescription to get homoeopathic remedies and you can buy these across the counter in many pharmacies and health stores. However, practitioners point out that it takes a great deal of skill and experience to choose the correct one for a given situation, as their diagnostic procedure not only takes into account the nature of the symptoms but also the patient as a whole.

Evidence of how varied the remedies are for different forms of essentially the same ailment can be found if you look in *The Prescriber*, which is a kind of mini-Bible listing the main homoeopathic preparations. For example, under the heading 'constipation' you'll find many different suggestions according to whether the sufferer is sedentary, has fainting fits, is subject to skin eruptions, experiences sinking feelings at the pit of the stomach, has hot flushes to the head, and so on for a list covering three pages. An equal amount of space is devoted to diarrhoea and the recommended treatment will vary depending upon, among many other factors, whether there is loss of confidence, a feeling of weakness after evacuation, or if it happens shortly after meals or perhaps only in the daytime, etc. With such a multitude of choices, selecting the right one is clearly a matter for the expert.

You can get more information about homoeopathy from: *The British Homoeopathic Association*, 27a Devonshire Street, London W1N 1RJ; *The Hahnemann Society*, Hahnemann House, 2 Powis Place, Great Ormond Street, London WC1N 3HT; *The Society of*

Homoeopaths, 2 Artizan Road, Northampton NN1 4HU.

AROMATHERAPY

The basic principle underlying this form of treatment is the use of essential oils – derived from wild or cultivated plants, herbs, fruits and trees – to restore the body's natural functions and rhythms. The essences are prepared so that they can be used in many different ways: as compresses, in baths, as inhalants, and for massages.

Practitioners claim that aromatherapy can help IBS sufferers in two major ways: either by using the essences directly to treat the gut, or using them as a way to control tension, anxiety and stress.

A word of caution is, however, in order: some of the oils used in aromatherapy can in fact be poisonous in other than the very smallest amounts and it is therefore absolutely essential that this therapy is administered under the supervision of a qualified person. You can get more information about aromatherapy from: *International Federation of Aromatherapists*, Department of Continuing Education, Royal Masonic Hospital, London W6 0TN; *The International Society of Professional Aromatherapists*, 41 Leicester Road, Hinckley LE10 1LW; *The Tisserand Association of Holistic Aromatherapy*, 65 Church Road, Hove, East Sussex BN3 2BS; or *The Register of Qualified Aromatherapists*, 52 Barrack Lane, Aldwyck, Bognor Regis, West Sussex PO21 7DD.

REFLEXOLOGY

In some ways the principle behind reflexology is quite similar to that of acupressure, except that in this instance the pressure is usually only applied to either the feet or the hands to create favourable changes elsewhere and also to stimulate the body's own ability to overcome disease by healing itself. The rate of success varies greatly, but the therapy is unlikely to be harmful and has been said to have been found effective by many who suffer from IBS.

According to reflexologists, different parts of the soles of the feet correspond to various parts of the gut and by stimulating the nerve endings in the right places on the feet they can improve the functioning of the organs of the digestive system. You could try reflexology on your own, but if the treatment tempts you then it's probably best to be shown how to use it by someone who has studied it in depth.

You can get more information from: *The British School of Reflexology*, 92 Sheering Road, Old Harlow, Essex CH17 0JW; *The Association of Reflexologists*, 110 John Silkin Lane, London SE8 5BE; *The Reflexologists' Society*, 39 Prestbury Road, Cheltenham, Glos GL52 2PT; or *The British Reflexology Association*, Monks Orchard, Whitbourne, Worcs WR6 5RB.

NATUROPATHY

Also known as 'naturopathic medicine', naturopathy is a broadly-based system that combines a wide variety of natural therapeutic and healing techniques and it can perhaps be best described as a mixture of traditional folk wisdom and modern medicine. The main underlying principle of this therapy is that the root-cause of all disease is the accumulation of waste products and toxins within the human body, this usually being the result of a lifestyle that is 'deficient'.

Naturopaths also believe that the human body has the wisdom and the power to heal itself, providing that we enhance rather than interfere with this power. As far as actual treatments are concerned, naturopathy relies heavily on herbal preparations and diet management techniques, the latter, of course, being particularly likely to be relevant for the relief of various IBS symptoms. The therapies that a naturopath may have to offer can include the following: physiotherapy, based on water, ultrasound, heat and cold; yoga or breathing exercises; biofeedback techniques; corrective nutrition; as well as some others, depending upon their training.

The naturopathic system of treatment relies heavily upon the practitioner and the patient discussing and agreeing upon what therapies to use. It also usually emphasises the promotion of psychological health and the benefits of stress reduction. Generally, this is an alternative therapy that has a good track record in helping IBS sufferers, especially those whose symptoms originate from tension and/or anxiety.

You can get more information from: *The General Council and Register of Naturopaths*, Frazer House, 6 Netherhall Gardens, London NW3 5RR; or *The Natural Therapeutic and Osteopathic Society and Register*, 14 Marford Road, Wheathampstead, Herts AL4 8AS.

BACH FLOWER REMEDIES

Dr Edward Bach was a noted homoeopathic physician and bacteriologist who created the Flower Remedies in the 1930s to treat 'emotional imbalances'. Although the remedies were originally formulated primarily to supplement homoeopathic preparations, they have since been used for all kinds of problems. Similar to the Flower Remedies – of which there are 38 kinds, all formulated by Dr Bach – are the Flower Essences which were developed later by other people following the guidelines laid down by Dr Bach.

Although most of the evidence about the efficacy of these remedies is purely anecdotal, many IBS sufferers have been reported as finding them helpful in reducing both the severity and frequency of symptoms. The remedies are available without prescription in many health shops, but once again it's a question of choosing the right one and it is therefore best to seek the advice of a qualified practitioner in the first instance.

You can get more information from: *The Edward Bach Centre*, Mount Vernon, Sotwell, Wallingford, Oxon OX10 0PZ.

HYPNOSIS AND HYPNOTHERAPY

These are two forms of treatment that are used quite commonly by conventional medicine as well as by alternative practitioners. The effects of hypnosis are well documented and, as described in Chapter

9 of this book, have given very good results in treating IBS patients whose symptoms had been refractory until then. There is, of course, a difference between the use of hypnosis by medical doctors or as it may be practised by someone whose qualifications are not as sound, so it's particularly important that you choose your hypnotherapist with great care.

Both hypnosis and hypnotherapy rely essentially on the power of suggestion, whether this suggestion comes from the therapist or from the patient themself. This kind of approach has proven particularly effective in treating the so-called 'psychosomatic' conditions, such as skin disorders, certain kinds of asthma, migraine, as well as certain types of IBS.

You can get more information from: *The British Society of Hypnotherapists*, 37 Orbain Road, Fulham, London SW6 7JZ; *The International Association of Hypnotherapists*, 1 Lowther Gardens, Bournemouth, Dorset BH8 8NH; *The World Federation of Hypnotherapists*, Belmont Centre, 46 Belmont Road, Ramsgate, Kent CT11 7QG; *The Professional Association of Hypnotherapists*, Natural Therapy Centre, Woodlands Road, Blaigowrie, Scotland PH10 6LD; *The National Council of Psychotherapists and Hypnotherapists Register*, 46 Oxhey Road, Oxhey, Watford, Herts WD1 4QQ; *British Hypnosis Research*, 8 Paston Place, Brighton, East Sussex BN2 1HA; *The Association of Holistic Hypnotherapists*, 17 Sycamore Close, Feltham, Middlesex TW13 7HN; or *The National Register of Hypnotherapists and Psychotherapists*, 12 Cross Street, Nelson, Lancashire.

YOGA

This is a well-known discipline that broadly speaking divides into two separate yet closely-linked components: first, there's a series of static or stretching exercises as well as breathing exercises; secondly, there is a meditation discipline that aims to help the subject reach a state of peace and harmony in the inner self.

At the physical level, yoga has proven itself to be extremely effective as a way of reducing stress levels and as such may often be of great help in dealing with the symptoms of IBS when these stem at least partly from psychological difficulties. As explained previously in Chapter 9 of this book, the meditation techniques can also be adapted to help those suffering from stress.

Although nearly all yoga exercises are considered to be safe for a moderately fit person, there are some that do initially create a great deal of strain on the back and the abdomen and as such should perhaps be avoided by IBS sufferers. All but the simplest yoga exercises should in any case only be undertaken under the supervision of a qualified teacher. It's also recommended that you should check with your doctor whether they think this is an advisable thing to do in your case.

You can get more information from: *The British Wheel of Yoga*, 1 Hamilton Place, Boston Road, Sleaford, Lincolnshire NG34 7ES; or *The Yoga for Health Foundation*, Ickwell Bury, Northill, Biggleswade, Beds SG18 9EF.

OSTEOPATHY

This is another alternative therapy that often finds great acceptance from the medical profession as a whole. The best way to find a good practitioner might well be to ask your doctor who could perhaps suggest someone in your area.

Developed in 1874 by Andrew Taylor Still, osteopathy has been found to be very effective in the relief of many stress-induced ailments. Based upon the underlying principle that 'structure governs function', osteopathy relies greatly on manipulative techniques which are addressed to the back and the neck. To treat IBS symptoms, the manipulation may also be extended to the spine and the abdomen. Although osteopathy can be very helpful, it can also be a dangerous form of treatment if administered by an inexperienced or unqualified person who may end up doing more harm than good. It's therefore vital that you should find a reputable and skilful practitioner.

You can get more information from: *The Register of Osteopaths*, 21 Suffolk Street, London SW1Y 4HG; or *College of Osteopaths Practitioners' Association*, 1 Furzegill Road, Borehamwood, Herts WD6 2DG.

IRIDOLOGY

This is in the first instance a diagnostic technique which divides the iris of the eye into 12 sections and relates each of those sections to specific parts of the human body. The iridologist analyses the information gleaned from their examination of the irises and uses this to spot health risks and provide an in-depth profile of the patient's overall healthcare needs. This information could, of course, be useful to IBS sufferers who believe their condition to be the result of more general health problems.

You can get more information from: *National Council and Register of Iridologists*, 40 Stokewood Road, Swinton, Bournemouth BH3 7NC; or *The Hale Clinic*, 7 Park Crescent, London NW1N 3HE.

HERBALISM

This is perhaps the oldest form of medicine and its history goes back at least 3,000 years to ancient China. Also known as 'herbal medicine', herbalism includes the use of various plant parts – root, bark, stem, flowers, leaf and even seeds – in different preparations for either internal or external use.

There has always been a strong association between herbal remedies and digestive problems. Even today Chinese physicians are often also trained in this branch of alternative medicine which takes into account not only the nature of the disease but also the personality of the patient.

Herbal remedies for digestive symptoms can be formulated in a wide variety of ways: as teas, potions, bath additives, juices, extracts, salves, lotions and ointments. There is, however, once again a need for a word of caution: some herbal preparations can be just as powerful – and therefore also potentially as toxic – as modern day drugs. So these remedies have to be prescribed and used with great care as they can create powerful side-effects, including dizziness, giddiness, indigestion and even more serious ones. It is essential therefore that herbal remedies should be prescribed by and used under the supervision of a suitably qualified medical herbalist.

You can get more information from: *The National Institute of Medical Herbalists*, 9 Palace Gate, Exeter, Devon EX1 1JA; *The National School of Herbal Medicine*, Bodle Street Green, Hailsham, East Sussex BN27 4RJ; or *The General Council and Register of Consultant Herbalists*, Grosvenor House, 40 Seaway, Middleton-on-Sea, West Sussex PO22 7SA.

The alternative therapies described above are, of course, only a small selection from the dozens of different ones available. While the mention of a therapy doesn't mean its endorsement, neither should the absence of such a mention be taken as indicating anything other that it has been left out either for reasons of space or because not enough creditable information about its use in the treatment of IBS was available.

Having said that, it is known that the following therapies and disciplines have been used at one time or another with varying degrees of success to provide relief from the symptoms of IBS.

THE ALEXANDER TECHNIQUE. The prime purpose of this training programme is to overcome poor habits of posture and movement and thereby reduce both physical and mental tension and reduce reaction to stress. Training in the technique – which was devised by an Australian actor, Fredrick Matthias Alexander – takes the form of a series of lessons in which the teacher guides the pupil to 'experience' their innate posture, movement and balance, which, according to Alexandrian teachings, become 'lost' or distorted by accumulated stress. Further lessons are also said to provide 'inspiration for deeper changes' and improvements in body-mind functioning. You can get more information from: *Society of Teachers of the Alexander Tech-*

nique, London House, 266 Fulham Road, London SW10 9EL; or *The Professional Association of Alexander Teachers*, Madian, Iorwerth Avenue, Aberystwyth, Dyfed SY23 1EW.

AUTOGENIC TRAINING AND THERAPY. This consists of a series of exercises which aim to generate a state of both mental and physical relaxation. It also includes some aspects of self-hypnosis in which the subject uses their own mind power to send themself positive, healing messages about their condition. It is a 'mind over matter' therapy that straddles the border between hypnosis and meditation, both of which, of course, are altered mind states. Many sufferers from IBS have reported autogenic training as being helpful to them, both as far as dealing with the symptoms of the syndrome and the stress factor which caused them were concerned. You can get more information from: *The British Association for Autogenic Training and Therapy*, c/o St John's Hospital, Stone, Aylesbury, Bucks; or *The Positive Health Centre*, 101 Harley Street, London W1 1DF.

Then there are the techniques which depend upon faith – not even necessarily the faith of the subject but quite often rather that of the practitioner:

HEALERS. There are literally dozens of different kinds of 'healing' techniques – including amongst many others, clairvoyant diagnosis, faith healing, laying on of hands, psychic healing, spiritual healing and energy healing. Healers have, of course, been credited with 'curing' all sorts of diseases and ailments, including IBS. But generally there is precious little objective evidence to back up these claims, although it must be accepted that merely being told 'you're feeling better' by someone in whom you have faith can indeed bring a positive, albeit frequently a temporary, improvement.

THERAPEUTIC TOUCH. Like some of the healers, practitioners of this therapy use a laying on of hands technique, but this is however not cloaked in mysticism and is free of any belief in supernatural forces. Instead it is described as being based on 'human energy transfer in the act of healing' and is intended for use by non-psychics.

It goes without saying that the success – real or imagined – of many alternative therapies relies heavily upon the link between mental and physical well-being. Conventional medicine also accepts the existence of this link and that it can have a profound influence on how patients may respond to treatments and how the course of a disease may progress. Whether any of the alternative therapies outlined above are likely to be helpful in your case is an individual decision you must make for yourself. Certainly some have helped many; the track record of others is however more patchy. Perhaps the single most important question to ask yourself is: Do you believe that they could help you?

Chapter 12

The Role Of Diet In Irritable Bowel Syndrome

A S MIGHT be expected, because Irritable Bowel Syndrome is a collection of symptoms that affect the digestive system, one of the main ways of dealing with it is by paying attention to what kind of foods you eat and how these may affect you.

Not only can the right kind of diet help reduce the severity and symptoms of IBS, it can also be a preventative measure which may stop the disorder from eventually afflicting those who might otherwise have been susceptible to developing it sooner or later.

There's an oft-quoted phrase 'You are what you eat' and while there is a great deal of truth in it, it by no means tells the whole story because it should be amended to 'You are what you eat and what your body can digest and then absorb for its use'. This is so because, after all, the main purpose of eating is to provide the right kind of nourishment for the body's various needs, not merely to satisfy the appetite, which after all is only the stimulant to get you to want to eat in the first place.

Merely eating an adequate and balanced diet is by no means always enough to provide the body with what it needs because, for example, the most nourishing and balanced food will only provide a limited amount of nutrition if for one reason or another it doesn't spend enough time in the digestive system to allow its nutrients to be fully absorbed. In addition, the body's request for food transmitted via the sensation of hunger or emptiness isn't always fulfilled because there's a Catch-22 situation that sometimes occurs in which the symptoms of IBS may make a sufferer so aware that certain foods may provoke symptoms that they even start to avoid eating; this avoidance may even include those foods which don't create discomfort or pain.

Essentially, there are three main aspects regarding diet that an IBS sufferer should consider:

1) How to maintain proper nutrition without creating IBS symptoms.
2) How to identify those foods that will actually help reduce the symptoms if you already have them in the first place.
3) How to seek out the foods that will prevent the symptoms from occurring.

There's also a fourth factor which needs to be taken into account because it has been shown that for some sufferers their symptoms are the result of food intolerance or allergy. What makes the situation even more complicated is that a food which may be guilty of provoking IBS in one patient may well be the very thing that another one can eat without any problem whatsoever. This is hardly surprising when you consider the wide range of different IBS symptoms. Quite logically one would expect the dietary approach to be different when dealing with someone whose main symptom is constipation as compared with another who suffers from severe diarrhoea.

Yet, although it would seem that different symptoms of IBS would call for different diets, this is not always the case and one of the most popular of diets for sufferers from IBS is the same whether indeed constipation or diarrhoea – or even both at varying times – are part of the clinical picture. This 'something for everyone' diet is one that is based on providing a very high amount of fibre which, according to most experts, speeds up the time it takes for food to travel through the digestive system.

Just how much a high fibre diet may do for you is a question of 'try it and see' because the accumulated clinical evidence can be confusing and even contradictory. The emphasis on fibre really started in this country some 20 years ago on the basis of the extremely good results obtained in one trial which studied the effects of an increased intake of bran by 30 IBS sufferers of whom 23 – that's a staggering three out of four – reported substantial improvement in their symptoms. Other studies later also brought similar but not quite so good results. When the researchers changed their attention from looking purely at bran as an additive to a normal diet and focused upon other diets that were equally rich in fibre generally, they found that these also helped many.

Good though it may be for some, a diet that's high in fibre content is by no means beneficial for all IBS sufferers and some have even found that it can make their symptoms worse. There's no magic test that you can take beforehand to find out whether or not you might gain from such a diet, but there's a pretty good chance that you might feel the better for it, the odds being more or less two to three in your favour. If it doesn't work out too well in your particular case after giving it a good try – having, of course, first consulted your doctor about it – you really won't have lost a great deal either.

THE HIGH FIBRE DIET

First of all, it's important to realise that the 'fibre' referred to is dietary fibre, which, as you may recall from reading in Chapter 7, is defined as being that part of a plant which cannot be digested by enzymes or acids in the human digestive system. This means, by definition, that only foods originally derived from plants are going to contain this fibre in the first instance. As a rule of thumb, you can also assume that the less the original food has been refined or processed before you eat it, the greater the amount of dietary fibre content there is likely to be.

Here to help you plan your diet are a few examples of the dietary fibre content of some common foods expressed as grams of fibre per 100 grams of the food:

Bread: brown, 5.1; white, 2.7; wholemeal, 8.5.

Cereals: muesli, 7.4; porridge, 0.8; puffed wheat, 15.4; shredded wheat, 12.3.

Biscuits: rye crispbread, 11.7; digestive, 5.5.

Vegetables (all boiled unless stated otherwise): tinned baked beans, 7.3; Brussels sprouts, 2.9; cabbage, 2.5; carrots, 3.1; cauliflower, 1.8; celery, 2.2; peas (originally frozen), 12.0; potatoes (baked/old), 2.5; potatoes (boiled/new), 2.0; fried chips (whether originally frozen or not), 3.2; spinach, 6.3; tinned sweetcorn, 5.7.

Fruit: peeled apples, 2.0; dried apricots, 24.0; bananas, 3.4; dried figs, 19.5; oranges, 2.0; peaches, 1.4; pears, 1.7; dried prunes, 16.1.

Nuts: almonds, 14.3; dessicated coconut, 23.5; peanuts, 8.1.

It's fairly obvious from the above league table that one of the easiest ways to increase your fibre intake is by substituting some of the foods you may be having currently for other similar ones which provide more fibre. So if you're a great consumer of bread, switch to the wholemeal variety; if you like vegetables, make sure that peas are often on the menu; and consider dried apricots or figs as an alternative to other fruit for dessert.

For those who have a breakfast cereal most days, this is one area where you can really boost your fibre intake without going to too much trouble by simply switching your current favourite for one of the bran-rich brands, such as *All-Bran* (dietary fibre: 30.0 per cent); *Bran Buds* (28.2 per cent); *Farmhouse Bran* (18.0 per cent); *Bran Flakes* (17.3 per cent); or *Sultana Bran* (15.5 per cent).

While it may not be all too difficult to increase fibre intake, the question also arises: how much is enough? There is some difference of opinion amongst experts on this one. For example, the *Committee on Medical Aspects of Foods* is on record as suggesting that the dietary fibre intake for a healthy adult should be 40 grams a day while the *National Advisory Committee on Nutrition Education* recommended 30 grams. To put these two different figures into perspective, it has been estimated that the current average adult intake is about 20 grams, so it's really a question of eating one and half times to twice as much of it for most people. Incidentally, it's also generally recommended that you shouldn't overdo things by eating much more bran too suddenly, but that you should increase your intake quite gradually over a fairly long period of time. Misplaced enthusiasm that manifests itself by changing to a diet that's too rich in fibre or not giving the body time to adjust to your new diet can in itself produce problems. So, the word from the experts is: increase your fibre intake, but do so slowly over a period of weeks and don't overdo things.

There are, of course, all sorts of scientifically worked out diets available from a variety of sources in which each last morsel of food has to be carefully weighed to match an equally carefully calculated table of ideal requirements. While that sort of thing may be useful for nutritionists or dieticians, it is less so under the circumstances that prevail in the normal family kitchen where each bit of food isn't placed on a scale and a note made of its contents. Most people can, however, quite easily achieve a diet that's high enough in dietary fibre by simply using their common sense to search out those foods which provide a lot of it and eating less of those which are poor in it.

Apart from increasing the fibre content of your food intake, there are some other recommendations about dieting that most experts agree may help ease some of the symptoms of IBS. Please note that the word 'some' is used to qualify experts in the previous sentence as opinions do vary considerably and it's virtually impossible to find a single facet of any aspect of IBS where everyone is in complete agreement. The following guidelines are, however, broadly speaking representative of the views shared by the majority.

TEA AND COFFEE. As you might have expected, these are on the 'avoid excessive intake' list for all sorts of reasons, one of the main ones being that caffeine – which is to be found in both tea and coffee – stimulates bowel action and therefore is less than indicated if diarrhoea is one of your symptoms. Another reason why it might be a good thing to curtail these drinks is that they can contribute to nervousness and tenseness, both of which can in turn lead to certain IBS symptoms.

FAT. That, too, is on the list of things that ideally you should avoid, particularly if one of your IBS symptoms is that of pain after meals as this could be the result of too much *cholecystokinin* being released and over-stimulating the colon. Cholecystokinin is a hormone secreted by the cells of the duodenum when it's filled with partly digested food, in particular fat. The hormone makes the gall-bladder contract and expel bile into the intestine where it stimulates the production of digestive enzymes by the pancreas. And over-production of this can lead to discomfort.

The main source of fat, of course, for many people is meat which on the average provides about a quarter of the total amount. The advice here is to switch to poultry or fish as much as you can and when you do have red meat, go for the leanest cuts you can find.

Another likely culprit in the fat stakes is cheese with some types, such as Cheddar, containing a whopping 34 per cent of it. The advice is choose carefully, taking the fat content into account. For example, nearly half of cream cheese is fat whereas cottage cheese has just one per cent of it. You'll also find 'traditional' cheeses with specially reduced fat contents on the shelves of most supermarkets.

Here are some other ways to reduce your fat intake: choose skimmed or semi-skimmed instead of whole milk; go for low-fat yoghurts; pick a polyunsaturated margarine instead of butter; try to steer clear of cakes, pastries and biscuits, most of which have quite a high fat content.

ALCOHOL. According to most experts, alcohol also finds itself if not on the 'strictly forbidden' list at least on the one that's headed 'avoid as much as reasonably possible', because it has been found that the cup that cheers can interfere with the absorption of nutrients. On the other hand, there is a small minority of dieticians who feel that the beneficial effects of a drink or two taken now and then, as the phrase has it, 'in moderation', may actually be helpful for some subjects. So, if giving up alcohol completely seems altogether too daunting to you, perhaps try easing off somewhat if you're currently anything more than a 'very moderate' drinker.

As you'll recall, we began this chapter by listing the three main aims of a dieting programme, these being to maintain proper nutrition while at the same time increasing your intake of foods which would either help you control or avoid your IBS symptoms and these aspects have now been covered by the guidelines above. There was, however, a fourth factor....

FOOD INTOLERANCE

While there are many foods which are recommended to help control the symptoms of IBS, the list of those which at one time or another have been identified as making things worse is virtually endless with just about anything edible having been implicated by sufferers.

Here's just a few of the things that some IBS patients have reported as causing painful digestion: onions, fried chicken, strawberry gateau, cauliflower, pork sausages, drinking chocolate, and so on and on. This, however, doesn't mean that just because these foods have worsened the symptoms for some patients that they will necessarily do so for others, as what your digestive system will deal with without a murmur varies considerably from individual to individual. Of course, what matters is what foods *your* digestive tract either finds acceptable or reacts to badly.

Obviously, in many instances, you'll know who the culprits are in your case. For example, if your IBS symptoms invariably start up after you've had a curry, you'll soon have made the connection and quite sensibly have dropped curries from your menu. But the situation is by no means always that clear-cut and it can sometimes take a bit of detective work to find out which foods really don't agree with you – or perhaps that should be the other way around and be 'which foods you don't agree with', because that's really the key question: what food is unsuitable for your highly individual digestive system?

There are essentially two basic ways to find out. The first – and perhaps by far the easiest of these – is simply to keep a diary of what you eat on a given day together with a note of your symptoms. Do this for a week or so and then look back and see if there is any easily spotted correlation between the two, such as a pain in the tummy the morning after each evening when you had chicken for dinner. When looking for these connections, bear in mind that there can be a substantial period of time separating the cause – that is the intake of the food under suspicion – and the resulting event in the form of IBS symptoms and that this time-lag may well be as much as three days or even more.

The other way to find out if certain foods are the cause of your problem is by excluding them from your diet and seeing whether that makes you feel better. This approach is more demanding and time-consuming, but it is much more likely to yield results.

Once again, when doing this, you should keep a diary in which you record both the excluded foods and your symptoms during the length of the experiment. You might be forgiven for believing that there really isn't any need to go to all this trouble, but memory can be fickle at the best of times and the only certain way to find out whether an exclusion diet is working or not is to have a fixed frame of reference against which you can compare it.

When you believe that you've identified a food – let's say, for example, white bread – whose elimination from your daily diet has seemed to have brought about an improvement in your symptoms, then it's worth double-checking that theory by deliberately reintroducing it for a few days to see if it makes things worse again. If the reintroduction of a suspect food causes the symptoms to come back, then you can be pretty sure that it is indeed a culprit.

While it's possible for someone to be intolerant of almost any food, there are some which time and time again have been shown to worsen the symptoms of IBS and therefore should be high on the list of those you test first. These offending foods frequently identified by others include: wheat products, particularly in a refined rather than in the 'whole' form; other kinds of foods derived from grain, such as oats or rye; any kind of very fatty or deep fried food, such as fish and chips; fruits with a sharp, strong taste, such as those of the citrus variety in particular; some ingredients of salads, including radishes, onions, cucumber, although lettuce is not likely to be an offender; and, as mentioned before, tea, coffee and alcohol.

Other foods that are likely to bring problems are dairy products and this includes not only the obvious ones like milk, cheese and yoghurt, but also many convenience foods which may include various ingredients derived from milk, such as whey, milk solids and skimmed milk powder.

Meat, as has been suggested earlier, and especially red meat, is another food that is likely to create difficulties so this should also be one of the items to be tested as part of your exclusion diet.

Naturally enough, it's obvious that to set out on a diet which wouldn't include any of the above would be extremely restrictive, if not just about impossible. And there's little point in setting out on an exclusion diet which is so limited that it's bound to fail in its objective. Instead, the approach recommended by most dieticians is that you eliminate a few of the suspect foods at a time and see whether that brings good results. For example, you may start off initially on a diet that only excludes the following: white bread, red meat, coffee and tea. If that doesn't help after a reasonable length of time, add some additional foods – such as milk and cheese – to the forbidden list, but if need be put back some of the foods you had eliminated originally to maintain a varied and acceptable menu. By first excluding a food for a while and then adding it back to your diet if it hasn't been found guilty, you can gradually work your way through all the likely suspects without being subjected to a diet that is so stringent and demanding that it becomes a source of stress.

There is another aspect of food intolerance which you may have to take into account. That is the fact that many dieticians believe that quite frequently the problems arise not just because of the intake of just one food but because two or more quite separate ones combine unfavourably to produce an adverse reaction. For example, red meat by itself may not cause you problems, but if you have white bread at more or less the same time, the two together may set off IBS

121

symptoms. If you have reason to believe that such a combination of foods may be the root-cause of your problems, then one of the ways to check this out is to grit your teeth and for a limited period eliminate all likely culprits from your diet. Should this rather drastic approach bring satisfactory results, you can gradually add back some of the suspect foods – one or two at a time – to your diet until the symptoms begin to get worse. When that happens, the chances are that one of the last items you've started eating again is the guilty food, either on its own or by acting in combination with something else.

It must be admitted that tracking down what food may be precipitating your symptoms is by no means an easy task and to do it properly will take some time, together with a great deal of determination and perseverance on your part. The prize you're pursuing – freedom from the pain and discomfort of IBS – is however certainly worth the trouble, as many former sufferers who managed to eliminate their symptoms this way would happily testify.

Finally, three notes of caution:

1) Don't be too ambitious in your exclusion programme by eliminating too many different foods at a single time. Just cut out two or three at a time – at the most, maybe four – and see you how get along. If that doesn't do the trick, don't give up, but go on to the next most likely suspects.

2) Ensure that you're still maintaining an adequate nutritional level while you're dieting and that you're getting enough of the various vitamins and minerals you need.

3) Do consult your doctor before dieting. Although it's unlikely, there could be reasons why they may advise you not to eliminate some foods for any length of time. If you're thinking of taking extra vitamins or mineral supplements to make up for those which you fear may be missing, also check this out first with your doctor as this, too, can be inadvisable under certain circumstances.

As a last thought, there's one approach to identifying what food may be harmful to you which doesn't have the benefit of scientific endorsement but is one that many IBS sufferers have said worked for them. The idea is very simple and consists of asking yourself 'What do I eat that I think may not be good for me?' The answer to that question can often be surprising and by no means obvious. If you try this and get a completely out-of-the-blue inspiration like, for example, 'liquorice', it's just worth a try giving up that item for a while and seeing if this makes any difference at all.

Chapter 13

Other Aspects Of
Irritable Bowel Syndrome

T HERE ARE quite a few other ailments or conditions which while
not specifically part of Irritable Bowel Syndrome are either often
associated with it or are confused with it until a full diagnosis has
been reached. In this chapter, we will look at these in some detail
and specially those whose symptoms can at times seem very similar
to those of IBS.

DIVERTICULOSIS

This is a condition in which small sacs or pouches have formed at
weak points in the alimentary tract. These sacs – called *diverticula*,
the singular form of which is *diverticulum* – can occur at almost any
point within the digestive system and include:

☐ **Pharyngeal diverticula** – These are to be found within the
pharynx and one of the likely symptoms is that the patient will
experience varying degrees of inflammation and pain on swallowing.

☐ **Oesophageal diverticula** – These occur in the gullet, that is the
middle or lower oesophagus. The cause, in this instance, is likely
to be a muscular disorder of the oesophagus although the condition
is usually symptom-free.

☐ **Gastric diverticula** – Once again these diverticula, which are to
be found in the stomach, don't usually provoke any symptoms.

☐ **Duodenal diverticula** – These form usually on the concave side of the duodenum and also usually don't create any noticeable symptoms. They are, however, frequently associated with indigestion which may take the form of pain or discomfort in the abdomen or lower chest region shortly after taking in food and this may be accompanied by either nausea and/or vomiting. Duodenal diverticula also carry an increased risk of *choledocholithiasis*, a condition in which stones occur in the common bile duct.

☐ **Jejunal diverticula** – They form in the small intestine where they may cause abdominal discomfort and also lead to poor food absorption because of the proliferation of bacteria within them.

☐ **Meckel's diverticulum** – This is a congenital abnormality which can occur in the ileum. It may become inflamed and provoke symptoms very similar to those of appendicitis or may lead to the formation of a peptic ulcer which in turn may give rise to pain, bleeding or perforation.

☐ Finally, there are **colonic diverticula** – whose symptoms are most likely to be confused with those of IBS – as they cause both abdominal pain as well as altered bowel habits. Additionally, they may become inflamed.

There are several terms used to describe various aspects of diverticular problems and it's just as well to be familiar with these so that should your doctor use them when making their diagnosis you will immediately understand them.

Diverticulitis means an inflammation of a diverticulum, although usually several diverticula are involved and most commonly those found in the colon. The cause of this is infection and it may well lead to pain in the lower abdomen which may be accompanied by constipation and/or diarrhoea. Diverticulitis could also cause an abscess to form and this may under certain circumstances require surgical drainage.

Diverticulosis merely describes the condition in which diverticula exist but where there is no inflammation and usually no symptoms.

Diverticular disease refers to the condition where, as above, there are diverticula, but these are not inflamed, but still provoke symptoms, such as pain in the lower abdomen and bowel habits which are disturbed. As there is no inflammation, the cause of the pain is usually spasm of the muscles of the intestine.

As you can see from the above, there are a great many different forms of diverticular problems. These can at times be mistaken initially for IBS and it has even been suggested that if the symptoms are only moderate a doctor may use the diagnoses of 'diverticular problems' and IBS somewhat interchangeably.

Treatment for diverticular disease can be quite similar to that for IBS in that antispasmodics, that is drugs that alter gut motility, may be used as well as bran supplements or bulk-forming laxatives. Should the diverticula in the intestinal wall become infected, then treatment is usually by antibiotics.

MYALGIC ENCEPHALOMYELITIS

Myalgic encephalomyelitis – which is better known simply by its initials as 'ME' or, more colloquially, as *post-viral fatigue syndrome* – is a disorder characterised by, amongst other symptoms, varying degrees of muscular fatigue and pain, slowness of movement, lack of concentration, possible loss of memory and extreme tiredness for no apparent reason. The cause of the disease has not as yet been fully established, but it has been associated with the presence of antibodies to enteroviruses – the latter being any virus that enters the body through the gastrointestinal tract, multiplying there, and then often invading the central nervous system. Common enteroviruses include:

Coxsackie viruses – of which there are about 30 different types. Type A Coxsackie viruses often cause diseases that are less severe and also not so well-defined, while Type B are frequently associated with inflammation or even degeneration of the brain, skeletal muscles or heart tissue.

Polioviruses – these are members of a small group of RNA-containing viruses that can cause poliomyelitis – which was once better known as 'infantile paralysis' or simply as 'polio'. Polio, of course, is rare in this country because of the high effectiveness of immunisation programmes in which either the oral Sabin vaccine or the injected Salk vaccine were used.

Rhinoviruses – these are also RNA-containing viruses, but they manifest themselves by causing respiratory infection symptoms that resemble those of the common cold.

As all these enteroviruses enter the human body via the digestive tract it is not surprising that they can also create some of the symptoms that are associated with IBS. There is another important similarity between ME and IBS in that both can create a very wide range of symptoms, some of which can at times appear conflicting. What's more, the symptoms of ME can also often wax and wane in intensity over a period of time as can those of IBS, this being one more reason why the two syndromes may be confused with each other. Naturally, it is also perfectly possible that someone may be unfortunate enough to have both IBS and ME at the same time.

Although enteroviruses are associated with ME, the exact cause of the syndrome continues to elude medical science. There are many theories, but precious few facts so far, although a considerable amount of research is being carried out at various medical centres, in particular at St Mary's Hospital in London.

Because of this lack of evidence as to the cause of ME, conventional medical treatment is therefore primarily addressed to dealing with its symptoms, with a highly variable degree of success. In fact, some doctors are not quite as sympathetic to ME sufferers as they might be because they believe that the syndrome may arise from a 'hysterical cause', that is one that originates in the mind and provokes all sorts of physical problems. Although it is now commonly accepted that ME is almost certainly the result of a virus that lingered on in the body long after it should have been dealt with, it must be said that there still are quite a few doctors who classify patients suffering from it as hypochondriacs, neurotics or even malingerers. It is perhaps because of this that many ME sufferers have turned to alternative practitioners for help.

Like IBS, ME can also be mistaken for a nervous illness as its many symptoms can include anxiety, depression and lethargy. Tranquillisers have at times been prescribed to treat these symptoms but they are often of little use and in some instances have even proven to be counter-productive.

There is no single clear-cut approach to treating ME, but it has been found that the majority of cases respond well to simple everyday measures such as getting enough rest, eating a diet that is both balanced and healthy, getting adequate fresh air and exercise, and keeping the bowel free from constipation as this helps restore the natural balance of the gut bacteria.

CANDIDA ALBICANS

Candida is a genus of yeast-like fungi – which was formerly known as *Monilia* – which inhabits the digestive tract as well as the vagina. One specific species – Candida albicans, which is a small oval-shaped budding fungus – is primarily responsible for causing an infection which can affect the mouth, the lungs, the intestine, the vagina, the skin and the nails.

The infection – called *candidiasis* and formerly known as *moniliasis* – is normally superficial in nature and occurs mainly in areas of the body that are usually moist, such as folds in the skin or the organs mentioned above. The popular term for candidiasis when it occurs in the mouth or the vagina is *thrush* and this use has extended over time even to describe the Candida albicans fungi itself.

Under normal circumstances, Candida albicans lives in the gut without causing any problems as the body's own defence mechanisms keep it under control. The difficulties start, however, when for one reason or another the fungus starts to proliferate in vast numbers. Just why that should happen isn't always clear, but these are just some of the causes that have been linked to Candida albicans reaching levels where it can become harmful:

☐ The use of certain medicines, including antibiotics, steroids, tranquillisers and some ulcer treatments, amongst others.

☐ The use of contraceptive pills.

☐ Somewhat paradoxically, the problems often follow a patient's complete or partial withdrawal from using either tranquillisers or sleeping pills when the difficulties usually reach their peak between six months and a year later.

☐ The wrong kind of food, 'wrong' in this context meaning that which is likely to feed the fungus rather than the person.

When the Candida albicans population grows to such an extent that the body can no longer keep it under control, two major developments can take place:

1) The fermentation process in the gut starts to become overactive with the result that a good deal more gas than usual is formed, this frequently leading to a bloated, distended abdomen. Hand in hand with this problem often come symptoms which are extremely similar to those of IBS, such as constipation, diarrhoea and changes in bowel habits.

2) The Candida albicans can change its form. In its original simple form it is limited to possibly causing thrush in the mouth or the vagina. When the yeast takes on its invasive form – which is characterised by tendrils sprouting from the cell – it can penetrate through the walls of the bowel and thereby create a route through which harmful substances can enter the bloodstream. Once this has happened, the whole body can be subjected to the assault of this form of chronic candidiasis and this may reflect itself in the appearance of many different kinds of symptoms. Apart from those which are also typical of IBS, these symptoms may include: acne, cystitis, infections in the ear or the nose, athlete's foot, skin rashes and bloating. In addition to these physical problems, chronic candidiasis is also linked to a gamut of nervous or psychological

difficulties, including heightened irritability, mental confusion, feelings of hopelessness, anxiety, distress and depression.

Conventional medical treatment for candidiasis is frequently in the form of *nystatin*, an antifungal drug. This can produce good results, but may take a while to do so, needing months rather than weeks to achieve a worthwhile effect. Nystatin may also unfortunately produce unwanted side-effects, the most commonly reported ones being nausea, vomiting and diarrhoea (the latter being particularly likely if the drug is prescribed at a high initial dosage). There is a further possible problem with this drug and that is that it can be too successful by killing off too much Candida albicans and this may lead to a condition known as a 'Herxheimer reaction', which simply means that you can feel generally unwell because there are too many poisons from the dead cells of the fungus in your system.

Another approach to treating candidiasis is by diet and there are many different suggestions as to what a sufferer should or should not eat. The most commonly used diet to reduce the Candida albicans population is based on excluding sugar in all its forms, as well as bread, cakes, biscuits, yeast products of any kind, most dairy products, fruit and fruit juices, and all foods or drinks containing citric acid, such as most tinned soups or tonic water. The diet also suggests that your consumption of whole grain foods should be restricted. If that makes you wonder what there is left to eat, the diet suggests the following as permissible: as many vegetables and salads as you want, potatoes in all forms, meat, chicken, fish, turkey, eggs, nuts, beans, as well as olive or sunflower oil.

Alternative treatments for reducing Candida albicans include eating crushed garlic cloves (these contain allicin, a powerful antifungal substance); consuming large quantities of live yoghurt; reducing your intake of caffeine and alcohol. Stopping smoking is also claimed to help.

EXCESS GAS

The normal gut produces something like two litres of gas each day and at any given moment about a fifth of a litre of it will be in the gastrointestinal system. Apart from the occasional burp or passing of wind, this gas doesn't usually present any problems. There are some people, however, whose production of gas is much higher than average and these unlucky people will be prone to suffer from either marked flatulence or belching. Although both of these symptoms are known collectively by the quite descriptive name of *burbulence*, the reasons for them – and the solutions to the problem – are quite different:

- ☐ Flatulence is the result of gas produced by bacteria in the large bowel and this usually reaches unacceptable levels when the resident bacteria in the gut are fed better than usual because their host has consumed foods that weren't capable of being digested fully by the enzymes in the small bowel, one such typical food being beans. The 'cure' – if that's the right word in this context – is usually simply avoiding those foods to which you know your digestive system will respond badly. Unfortunately, most of the high fibre foods – which are otherwise recommended for IBS sufferers – do also tend to create more gas so it may be a question of choosing the lesser of two evils.

- ☐ The gas released by belching, on the other hand, is usually the result of the subject having swallowed too much air while eating. While we all swallow some air, there are some – especially those of a nervous disposition – who take in a great deal more of it than normal and varying amounts of this will then reach the stomach from where most of it will have to be released in one direction or the other. Apart from the obvious suggestion that someone subject to belching would do well to avoid carbonated drinks, the other way to reduce the problem is by eating more slowly and swallowing food deliberately rather than gulping it down.

A LUMP IN THE THROAT

Most of us now and then get a feeling that is best described as 'a lump in the throat' in which the lump seems to take residence just below the back of the throat itself. Although the sensation may be mildly uncomfortable for a while, it usually goes away of its own accord. There are, however, some people – and IBS sufferers seem to be part of this group – who get a lump much more frequently than normal and when they do, it often hangs on seemingly forever.

Medicine has several possible explanations for this sensation:

☐ It could be due either to general physical or mental tension.
☐ It might be caused by one of the muscles in the back of the throat not relaxing fully after it had previously contracted, for example, after eating.
☐ The cause could be 'over-swallowing', that is swallowing rapidly several times in succession, leaving the throat deprived of sufficient saliva to lubricate it.

Whatever the real reason might be, a lump in the throat sensation – which incidentally has the rather frightening medical name of *globus hystericus* – is usually nothing to worry about. Should it happen frequently, or should you be at all concerned about it, it is nevertheless a good idea to consult your doctor about it.

A PAIN IN THE LOWER END

There is another common condition which although it may affect anyone at any time is, however, also more likely to occur in people who have IBS. Known as either *proctalgia* or *proctodynia*, it means having a pain in either the rectal or anal regions. There is a sub-form of this disorder called *proctalgia fugax* in which a severe pain suddenly strikes the rectum and this may last for just a few seconds, some minutes, or even an hour or so with attacks being separated by days, weeks or possibly many months.

The pain triggered by an attack of proctalgia fugax can be extremely intense, so strong that it may cause not only physical agony but also great worry as to what the underlying reason for it might be. Temporary relief may be attained by one or more of the following measures:

☐ Putting the body in a doubled up position by bringing the knees up towards the chest and clasping them with your hands.

☐ Applying cold or heat near the affected area.

☐ Gently massaging the muscles around the pain.

☐ Having a bowel movement, but without straining to produce one if it doesn't come easily.

☐ Taking a warm bath.

The exact cause of proctalgia fugax remains unknown although it appears likely that the pain is caused by a spasm in one or more of the muscles in the area where the rectum joins the anus.

Although there is no recognised medical treatment for proctalgia fugax – the condition isn't even listed in the *British National Formulary*, nor is it to be found in many medical dictionaries – you should still see your doctor if you're affected, if only so they can eliminate other possible reasons for the pain, such as pelvic disease or prostate problems.

HYPERVENTILATION AND IBS

Hyperventilation – the common term for which is 'overbreathing' – is the name given to breathing that is very rapid and shallow and makes use of the upper chest rather than the abdomen. Breathing for any length of time in this way usually produces some of the following three main effects:

1) It results in an over-production of oxygen which is produced in greater quantities than the body either needs or can utilise. This extra oxygen is matched by a reduction of the amount of carbon dioxide in the blood.

2) It alters the acid/alkaline balance of the body and this change can set off all kinds of strange, unusual and even frightening feelings, such as faintness, dizziness,

cramps, pain in the neck and shoulders, and – as might have been expected – digestive upsets.

3)   It is also likely to trigger off suddenly a strong feeling of breathlessness, and this in turn may well lead to so-called 'panic attacks', a condition in which the subject becomes overwhelmed by fear and apprehension for no obvious reason.

One of the reasons why hyperventilation is of particular relevance to IBS sufferers is that one of its causes can be an abdomen that is bloated and therefore cramps the lungs. This makes the subject breathe more with the chest and less with the abdomen so that hyperventilation may result and possibly trigger off panic attacks. Incidentally, should you have a panic attack, here are two good ways of dealing with the problem:

☐ Empty your lungs as much as is possible without causing discomfort by letting out a prolonged sigh. Then cup your hands loosely around your mouth and breathe in with your mouth. What happens when you do this is that you're breathing in once again some of the air you've just exhaled and this, being comparatively rich in carbon dioxide, will help restore the correct oxygen/carbon dioxide balance in your blood.

☐ An alternative way of obtaining the same effect is by placing a paper bag so that it loosely covers your mouth and nose and you breathe naturally in and out of the bag. Very soon, you will find that your breathing rate slows down and becomes normal once again. It must be stressed that you should never use a plastic bag for this and the paper bag you do use should just be held in place by your hands and not attached to your head in any way.

While the simple remedies suggested above may help you cope with hyperventilation during a bad attack of it, the long-term answer to the problem lies in doing exercises which teach you 'abdominal breathing'. Here's one such exercise:

First of all, either sit or lie down comfortably after having loosened any clothing that might restrict the throat, chest or abdomen. Put one of your hands on your abdomen and the other on your chest. As your breathing becomes more abdominal, you should feel that the hand on your abdomen rises slowly up and down to match your breathing cycle while the hand on your chest remains still.

When you breathe in, let the abdomen rise; when you breathe out, let it drop down again. Breathe slowly – something like around about ten times a minute – and do so through your nose, keeping your mouth closed.

To achieve results, this exercise should initially be carried out twice a day for about twenty minutes at a time. Later on, when your abdominal breathing has gone as it were on automatic pilot, you can reduce the number and length of exercise sessions.

THE COMPLETE HANDBOOK
OF
HEALTH TIPS

A NEW BOOK REVEALS VITAL Health Tips based on the latest nutritional and scientific findings and time-proven remedies. This book is of vital importance to everyone interested in their health. Here are a few tips covered in this *Complete Handbook of Health Tips*:

- How to get more energy and combat fatigue (2 nutrients may help).
- How to flatten your tummy with a 20 second, daily exercise.
- A nutrient that may help improve memory.
- How to deal with stress, including what nutrients may be helpful.
- A nutrient that may increase resistance to disease.
- 4 simple ways to take off weight.
- The only effective way to get rid of cellulite.
- 4 tips for relieving mouth ulcers.
- A cheese that can help prevent tooth decay.
- A herbal remedy to prevent migraine headaches.
- One doctor's way to prevent grey hair.
- How to get rid of facial hair.
- How to shorten miseries of a cold.
- 3 tips for relieving sinus congestion.
- 5 ways to stop foot odour.
- 3 nutrients to minimise harmful effects of alcohol.
- 2 vitamins that may help avoid bruises.

- 5 ways to relieve haemorrhoids.
- How to relieve nightly leg cramps.
- Prostate trouble: a simple tactic to alleviate getting up during the night.
- A nutrient that may help lower blood pressure.
- 4 tips to fall asleep faster.
- How to detect and relieve food allergies.
- A tip for preventing car sickness.
- How to prevent bladder infections.
- A vitamin that may repel insects when taken orally.
- A simple technique to relieve tension.
- How to relieve dry skin.
- 4 tips to avoid food poisoning
- How to stop snoring.
- 3 ways to avoid stomach irritation when taking aspirin.
- 4 vitamins that may be harmful if taken in excess.
- 6 aids to eliminate constipation.
- 7 suggestions to relieve heartburn.
- A safe, simple home treatment for sore, tired feet.
- How to relieve bloating and puffiness.
- A common food to reduce cholesterol.

You can order the book direct from the publisher and save. To order simply send £9.95 *(which includes postage and handling)*, together with your name, address and book title to: Carnell plc, Dept IBSH, Alresford, nr Colchester, Essex CO7 8AP. You can return the book at any time within three months for a full refund if not satisfied.